AF673422

VEDIC HEALTH CARE SYSTEM

Sushrut Sanhita is the epic of Shalya Chikitsa. The exact meaning of Shalya is the study of imbalance of four humors—Vat, Pitta, Kaph and Rakta—or disease produced by them, identification of disease or the method of curing the disease.

Siravedhan and Marm chikitsa were very prevalent and highly accepted therapy during Vedic period and these principles of therapy were available mainly in Rigved and Atharvaved and got flourished during Sanhita period.

The book endeavours to present *Sushrut Shalya Chikitsa,* which is almost lost today, in its simplest form so that it may give the right direction to the students and researchers of Ayurveda.

Vedic Health Care System

Clinical Practice of Sushrutokta Marm Chikitsa and Siravedhan

(Highlighting Acupuncture)

RAM LAL SHAH
BINOD KUMAR JOSHI
GEETA JOSHI

New Age Books
New Delhi (India)

VEDIC HEALTH CARE SYSTEM

Clinical Practice of Sushrutokta Marm Chikitsa and Siravedhan

ISBN: 978-81-7822-041-3

Reprint: Delhi, **2017**
Second Revised Edition: Delhi, 2005
First Edition: Delhi, 2002

Published by
NEW AGE BOOKS
A-44 Naraina Phase-1
New Delhi-110 028 (INDIA)
Email: nab@newagebooksindia.com
Website: www.newagebooksindia.com

Library of Congress Cataloging-in-Publication Data
Shah, Ram Lal; Joshi, Binod Kumar; and Joshi, Geeta
ISBN : 978-81-7822-041-3
Includes Foreword, Abbreviations,
Introduction,Glossary, Bibliography,
Index, Fig.Index
Ayurveda/Health

Printed and published by
RP Jain for New Age Books
A-44 Naraina Industrial Area
Phase-1, New Delhi 110 028, India

FOREWORD

It gives me great pleasure to write the foreword of this book "Vedic Health Care System: Clinical Practice of Sushrutokta Marm Chikitsa and Siravedhan". In the Vedic era, Siravedhanam and Agnikarma were practiced for treating a number of ailments. Ayurved, the Science of Indian medicines, while treating the patient, adopts a holistic approach. Siravedhan and Marm chikitsa were very prevalent and highly accepted therapy during Vedic period and these principles of therapy were mentioned in Rigved and Atharvaved and got flourished during Sanhita period. It is amazing to read the details of treatment which Sushrut described in Sushrut Sanhita. With no modern equipments available to those early physicians, the intricate description of Sira, Dhamani and Marm leave the best of todays minds wondering as to what force guided them to see through the patient and treat him with the best of results. We, in the present era, need to study the work of those early physicians and learn the practice of Siravedhanam and Agnikarma.

I am sure that after reading this book, the concept of Marm and Siravedhanam will be better understood and finally it will be clear to the whole world that Acupuncture as we understand today is one of the component of age-old Shalya Chikitsa and is the Indian study of Dhanvantari School.

I compliment authors of this book and wish them all the success in life and hope that this book will prove a boon for treatment of ailments and a guide for learners of Ayurveda be it a student or a practitioner or researcher in this field.

Dr. H.S. Sharma

Ex. Dean

- Institute of Post Graduate Teaching & Research Gujrat Ayurved University, Jamnagar, Gujrat
- *Ex Director* - Principal National Institute of Ayurved, Jaipur
- *Patron* - Aihore Pratisthanam Osaka Ayurveda Kenkyusho, Japan, Osaka

PREFACE TO THE SECOND EDITION

The scholars, learned intellectuals and the worthy readers are subject of thanks who accepted the first edition of *Vedic Health Care System* with great interest and enthusiasm. We are very happily encouraged to present the second edition with few corrections in view of the demand and exhaustion of the first edition in such a short period from the world market. We deem our labour in research as suitably rewarded as of the appreciation and encouragement received from different corners of the world.

It gives us great pleasure to be highly grateful to those valued researchers and intellectuals who really were not resisted to write back that this research of ours has cleared the doubt of thousand years of darkness and has put an end of all the misconceptions on the subject.

PREFACE TO THE FIRST EDITION

All that has been written in Vedas regarding health care system in general, Siravedhan and Agnikarm in particular can not be compiled in one book. Ayurved treats the patient as a whole. In other words one should have a holistic approach to treat a patient. In fact, Marm Chikitsa ensures better results when practised as a combination therapy of Ayurvedic care. For example while treating chronic pain by Siravedhan other aspects of health of the patient must be considered for better response.

Siravedhan and Marm chikitsa were very prevalent and highly accepted therapy during Vedic period and these principles of therapy were available mainly in Rigved and Atharvaved and got flourished during Sanhita period. Dhanvantari has elaborated these methods in a very simple and practical form in *Sushrut Sanhita.* Uses of herbs, animal products, minerals and metals by different scientific methods and surgical and para-surgical methods alongwith cure of ailments by patient's own body points were the main methods of treatment. During that period, treatment through Dhamani, Sira and Marm was in its supreme and highly developed. Gradually with the passage of time and regular outside invasions all Vedic literatures on Astrology, Grammer and Ayurved almost got faded in memory. Fixed misconceptions reigned and ruined the great science of Ayurved and non-availability of diagrams and illustrations were also responsible for this. This is the reason that even today Dhamani and Sira are wrongly interpretated as blood carrying Artery and Veins. An important question remained unanswered till today about the location of 24 Dhamanis and 700 Siras mentioned in *Sushrut Sanhita.* Calculations and distributions of 700 Siras alongwith calculations and distributions of 10 urdhva, 10 adhah and 4 tiryak Dhamanis are still unknown. While according to *Sushrut Sanhita Sutra Sthan* 14 and *Sharir Sthan* 9 it is the Rasa which flows in the Dhamani and not the blood. Sushrut has clearly mentioned in *Sharir Sthan* 9/ 4-9 and *Sutra Sthan* 14/3 that these 24 Dhamanis and 700 Siras are responsible for the control of Respiration, Urination, Defecation, Menstruation etc. and only these extract out (yapan) the disease. The body remains healthy and disease free because of the free and unobstructed flow of Rasa. Any obstruction on particular pathway of Rasa results in particular disease and can be rooted out by re-regulating the flow of Rasa by Siravedhan.

Then why and how blunder was committed of confirming Dhamani as Artery and Sira as Veins. Ailments like Asthma, fever, obstruction in urine etc. cannot be rooted out by Artery. Even today few words of Sushrut could not be understood in their right perspective and therefore it might have been the reason of not realising the power of rooting out the disease through Dhamani. The meaning of 'yapan' could not be translated and understood and has been in use as such till now. However the meaning of 'yapan' unfolds all the pages to understand the curing property of Sira, Dhamani and Marma because the meaning of 'yapan' is to extract out (root out) the disease.

Chinese literature of Acupuncture when decoded answers to it. In fact 24 channels (meridians) of Chinese Acupuncture are nothing else than Sushrut's 24 Dhamanis while points on channels are 700 Siras of Sushrut. Sushrut has very authentically mentioned that Siras are embedded in Dhamanis other than extra canals. Similarly, external Marmas are also composed of these Siras wherein bones, nerves, joints etc. also appear as per their specific locations. In fact this knowledge has already got passed to the nearby countries around India mainly during 'Buddha' period and got stored as in cold storage. It is not a coincidence that almost all Buddhist countries have this knowledge and it is the Indian fortune that the origin of this knowledge is from India.

Many unsolved and unanswered subjects of Chinese Acupuncture can be solved and understood comprehensively by *Sushrut Sanhita*. This work of ours may be of specific help in this direction. *Sushrut Sanhita* can now be understood in better perspective. Keeping this view the future researchers and translators would unfold still newer subjects and strengthen further the Ayurved and medical science. The detail description and method of treatment in the form of sutra shall help in eliminating the ailments of human being.

ABBREVIATIONS

Ama	: Amashay Dhamani
A.N.	: Artav Nadi
G.B.	: Gall Bladder Channel
H or Ht.	: Heart Channel
K	: Kidney Channel
Lagh	: Laghvantra Dhamani
LI	: Large Intestine Channel
Liv.	: Liver Channel
Lu.	: Lung Channel
Mutra	: Mutrashay Dhamani
P	: Pericardium Channel
Phuff	: Phuffus Dhamani
Pitta	: Pittashay Dhamani
S	: Sushrut
Shlesh	: Shleshmashay Dhamani
Shle	: Shleshmashay Dhamani
Sh. Chi	: Sushrut Sanhita Chikitsa sthan
SI	: Small Intestine Channel
Sj	: Sanjiao Channel
Sp	: Spleen Channel
S.N.	: Shukra Nadi
S. Su	: Sushrut Sanhita Sutra Sthan
S. Sh	: Sushrut Sanhita Sharir Sthan
Su. Chi	: Sushrut Sanhita Chikitsa Sthan
Su. Nidan	: Sushrut Sanhita Nidan Sthan
Su. Sha	: Sushrut Sanhita Sharir Sthan
Su. Sh.	: Sushrut Sanhita Sharir Sthan
St	: Stomach Channel
T. Hri	: Tal Hridaya
U.B.	: Urinary Bladder Channel
V.A.	: Vrihadantra Dhamani
Vrih	: Vrihadantra Dhamani
Vr	: Vrikka Dhamani
Yak	: Yakrit Dhamani

CONTENTS

INTRODUCTION

Sushrut Sanhita is the epic of Shalya Chikitsa. The exact meaning of Shalya is the study of imbalance of four humors Vat, Pitta, Kaph and Rakta or disease produced by them, identification of disease or the method of curing the disease.

According to Sushrut an uninterrupted circulation of the living factor Rasa (Chinese call it Qi) is responsible for a good health and any obstacle in the circulation results in disease. The disease appears in its true form in that channel where there is an obstruction. The disease is cured if the path or speed of circulation of Rasa is revived. This Rasa is circulated in the Dhamanis and there are seven hundred Siras embedded in these Dhamanis. The four types of Siras responsible for the circulation of *Vat, Pitta, Kaph* and *Rakta* are almost situated at the Marmas. Stimulation of these Marmas revives the circulation of Rasa in the Dhamanis.

Unfortunately meaning of Sira, Dhamani and Marmas has till now been wrongly translated because of which *Sushrut Sanhita* could not be understood in its right perspective. Sira has been misunderstood as vein, Dhamanis as artery and Marmas are mistakenly read as the tissues to be saved during surgery. In fact Sira and Dhamani are not vein and artery instead they are the pathways of the micro-element Rasa not visible by naked eye and can be seen by electronic instruments. Even Shushrut has said that the micro-refined Rasa flows through Dhamani and Sira and not the blood. Sira and Dhamani are not vein or artery instead they are the channels for the circulation of Rasa.

Except in a very few places Rakta Mokshan does not mean blood letting from the body, instead it means to revive the speed of circulation of blood in the channels. It is again to be made clear that during acupuncture the meaning of one Prastha Shonit Mokshan does not mean blood letting of 13.5 Pal of blood by weight instead it means the time factor involved for one Prastha shonit Mokshan. This is the time involved to stimulate the Sirabindu and it comes out to 13.5 minutes i.e. the Sirabindu is to be stimulated for 13.5 minutes.

We would like to make it clear here that Marmas, when affected cause disease mean that particular Marmas which are at Torso, extremities and head represent the vital organs of the body and by stimulating these outer points the disease can be cured.

For example, Kshipra Marmas which are situated at the extremities when punctured result into death, does not at all mean that when hands are affected it will result into death. Infact Kshipra Marmas at the extremities of hands and feet shows their being diseased or Viddha of that internal vital organs Marm and the disease can be rooted out from Kshipra Marma of extremities. According to Sushrut death occurs due to Akshep when Kshipra Marma is Viddha(Su.Sh.6/31.32).It must be made very clear here that Kshipra Marma is the marm related to blood coagulating system and this Marm is also related to the system of Akshep(Apoplexy).Thus when Kshipra Marma is Viddha (system affected by disease) - the disease occurs and it can be cured by stimulating the marm points of hands or feet. This is relevant for all the Marmas.

It pains to write that the *Sushrut Sanhita* has been translated so wrongly that at one place it is mentioned that when Kshipra Marma is viddha—cut the hands and feet from Manibandh which sounds very funny (*Sushrut Sharir,* 6/33 *Vimarsha* (comments)) Through this book our endeavour is to present *Sushrut Shalya Chikitsa,* which is almost lost today in its simplest form so that it may give the right direction to the students and, researchers of Ayurveda.

Chapter 1

DHAMANIS
(Channels and Meridians)

Dhamani are not the synonym of Arteries but Dhamanis are meridians or channels. According to *Sushrut Sutra Sthan,* 14/3:

तत्र पाञ्चभौतिकस्य चतुर्विधस्य षड्रसस्य
द्विविधवीर्यस्याष्टविधवीर्यस्य वाऽनेकगुणस्योपयुक्तस्याहारस्य
सम्यक्परिणतस्य यस्तेजोभूतः सारः परमसूक्ष्मः
स 'रस' इत्युच्यते, तस्य हृदयम् स्थानम्
सहृदयाच्चतुर्विंशतिधमनीरनुप्रविश्योर्ध्वगा
दश दशाधोगामिन्यश्चतस्त्रश्चतिर्यग्गाः
कृत्स्नं शरीरमहरहस्तर्पयति वर्धयति
धारयति यापयति चादृष्टहेतुकेन कर्मणा

(सु० सू० स्था०,14/3)

Tatra panch bhotikasya chaturvidhasya shadrasasya
dvividh veeryasyashtvidhveerayasya vaanekgunsyopyukta
syaharasya samyakparinatasya yastejobhootah
sarah paramsukshmah sa 'Ras' ityuchyate
tasya hridayam sthanam sa hridayachchaturvinshati
dhamani ranupravishyordhvaga dash dashadhogaminyashch-
tastrashchtiryaggah kritsnam shariramharhastarpayati
vardhayati dharayati yapayati chadrishthetuken karmana

(Su. Su. Sth. 14/3)

Again in *Sushrut Sharir,* 9/4-9, Acharya Sushrut says:

तासां तु खलु नाभिप्रभवाणां धमनीनामूर्ध्वगा दश,
दश चाधोगामिन्यः चतस्रस्तिर्यग्गाः।

उर्ध्वगाः शब्द रूप रस गन्ध प्रश्वासो --------
अधोगमास्तु वातमूत्र पुरीष ----------------
तिर्यग्गाणां तु चतसृणां धमनीनामेकैका शतधा
सहस्रधा-----तासां मुखानि रोमकूप प्रति बद्धानि-----।

(सु० शा०, 9/4-9)

Tasam tu khalu nabhiprabhavanam dhamaninam urdhvaga dash,
dash chadhogaminyah chatastrastiryaggah
urdhvagah shabda roop ras gandh prashvaso .....
adhogamastu vatmutra purish ......
tiryagganam tu chatasrinam dhamaninamekaika shatadha
sahatsradha ...... tasam mukhani romkup pratibaddhani.......

(Su. Sh., 9/4-9)

Above facts force us to be of the firm opinion that Dhamanis are not the vessels of blood circulation but these are the channels which govern the activities like perception, respiration, urination, defecation, anaesthesia etc. Book in Chinese Acupunture when decoded also confirms the same. So According to Sushrut there are twenty-four Dhamanis as shown below:

10 Ascending or Dhatu Dhamani
10 Descending or Ashaya Dhamani
4 Transverse or Tiryag Dhamani

The finest essence of four types of food that we take, flows through these Dhamanis and Chinese call it as Qi (Chi) and Acharya Sushrut calls it as Param Sukshma Rasa (ultramicroscopic live force) which is not detectable in cadaver. The presence of these meridians can also be judged by Anuman (perception) by the symptoms shown in the body because of the fullness or emptiness of these channels.

These channels are described under five Mahabhutas namely:

Akash	(Wood	= Liver and gall-bladder (G.B.))
Vayu	(Metal	= Lung and large intestine)
Tej	(Fire	= Heart and small intestine)
Jal	(Water	= Kidney and urinary bladder (U.B.))
Prithvi	(Earth	= Spleen and stomach)

Four Tiryag Dhamanis are: Talhridaya (Pericardium channel) and Shleshmashay (Sanjiao (Sj) channel).

Tiryag Dhamanis are without organ.

The function of Param Sukshma Rasa is to nourish the body continuosly all the 24 hours, as kidney meridian nourishes ears while gall bladder meridian nourishes eyes (see Shringatak Marm, *Su. Sharir*, 6/27). This Ras is responsible for growth, supports the live forces of the body and cures the diseases. This is essential for treatment. This function is under the subconscious level and cannot be measured objectively. According to Sushrut its mechanism of action cannot be consciously defined.

Chapter 2

DHAMANIS (CHANNELS) NOMENCLATURE

UPPER EXTREMITY

Lung Channel (Lu)—*Urdhvaga phuffus dhamani* (Figure 6)

It emerges as Lu 1 below the acromial extremity of the clavicle, descending along the medial aspect of the upper arm and ends as Lu 11 at the medial side of the tip of thumb. According to su. Uttar., 46/22:

नरवाभ्यन्तरतोत्रपातैः

(सु०उ०,46/22)

Nakhabhyantartotrapataih

(Sushrut uttar, 46/22)

Heart Channel (H)—*Urdhvaga hridaya dhamani* (Figure 10)

It emerges as H1 from the centre of the axilla and runs on the medial aspect of the upper arm and ends as H9 at the medial aspect of the tip of little finger.

Pericardium Channel (P)—*Talhridaya tiryak dhamani* (Figure 1)

It starts as P1 in the fourth inter costal space 1" lateral to the nipple, running over the centre of the palm ending at the tip of middle finger.

Large Intestine Channel (LI)—*Adhoga vrihdantra dhamani* (Figures 2, 7)

It starts from radial side of the index finger about 0.1 inch posterior (dakshin) to the corner of the nail, runs upward form the famous Kshipra Marm as LI4 and runs along the lateral side of the elbow. On reaching lateral side of the elbow it forms a part of Kurpar Marm, ascends to the highest point of the shoulder and has indication for important disease of motor impairment,'vishvachi'. In the upper aspect of Shoulder as L I 16 has the indication for Ansashosha and Avabahuk. There after it traverses on the lateral side of the neck ending in the nasolabial groove forming fan Marm.

Small Intestine Channel (SI)—*Adhoga laghvantra dhamani* (Figure 11)

Starts as SI1 from the ulnar side of the tip of the little finger, reaching wrist it forms the Manibandh Marm, ascends along the posterior aspect of the forearm from where it reaches the medial side of the shoulder joint as S I 10,11,12, having the indication for Ansashosha and Avabahuk. Finaly it ends as SI19 between the tragus and the mandibular joint having the indication for Vadhirya.

Sanjiao Channel (Sj)—*Tiryaga shleshmashay dhamani* (Figures 14,19)

Starts from the tip of ring finger as Sj1 running upward to form the Manibandh Marm at the wrist joint runs upwards as Sj10 at the posterior side of the elbow which is indicated in yakritodar. Reaching posterior part of the shoulder indicated in Vishvachi as Sj14, Traverse posterior the lobule of ear encircles to the ear lobule forming Vidhur Marm, as Sj17, 18, 19, 20, 21. Finally it ends in the depression at the lateral end of the eyebrow forming Apang Marm.

LOWER EXTREMITY

Spleen Channel (Sp)—*Urdhvaga pliha dhamani* (Figures 3, 5, 9)

It has total 21 points. It starts from the medial side of tip of big toe as Sp1. It runs along the medial side of foot reaching the knee joint as Sp9. Up to this point its element is earth (prithvi) Running upwards into the thigh reaches the inguinal groove as Sp12 and enters into the abdominal wall. Ascending upwards forming 3 very important Marmas as Stanrohit, Apastambha and Stanmool. Above the knee its element is Saman Vayu.

Liver Channel (Liv)—*Urdhvaga yakrit pittaj dhamani* (Figures 5, 13, 26)

Start from the lateral side of the great toe as Liv1 and reaching just above Liv3 it makes the famous Kshipra Marm with stomach Channel. Running upwards it passes through the medial malleolus and ascends upto the knee as Liv9 to form the Ani Marm. Up to this point its element is Akash and beyond it is fire reaching at inguinal groove it forms Vitap Marm. It enters the abdomen as Liv13 to form the front Mu point of spleen i.e. Dakodar yantra (Ubhaya Mukhi Nadi Yantra). Its last point is Liv14.

Kidney Channel (K)—*Urdhvaga vrikka kaphaj dhamani* (Figures 5, 16, 20)

It starts from the depression of the sole as K1 forming Talhridaya Marm and enters the heel below medial malleolus. Then it ascends along the medial side of the leg and in the calf muscle it runs by the side of Indrabasti Marm reaching the knee joint as K10. Then it goes upwards along the postero-medial aspect of thigh reaching the inguinal canal makes the Vitap Marm. Finally it enters the abdomen and goes upwards to chest ending in K27.

Stomach Channel (St.)—*Adhoga amashaya vataj dhamani* (Figures 2, 5, 8)

It start as St1 from the midpoint of the infra orbital ridge. Descends down to St 6 on the lower angle of the mandible, from here a branch runs upwards at St8 to form the Lalat Marm. The main trunk runs downwards from St6 on to the lateral part of the neck forming Neela, Manya Sira Marm Reaching one rib below the nipple as St18 it forms the stanmool Vaksha Marm Running downwards to St25 to form the front Mu point of large intestine (one of the Dakodar yantra) then it reaches superior to the inguinal groove as St30 with indication of vriddhi (Hernia). Reaching middle of the thigh at point St32 to form Urvi Marm and directly below is St33 as Ani Marm. It traverses downwards below the patella and lateral to the patellar ligament as St35 Janu Marm. The famous point St36 having the indication of Udar-Rog, Ardhangvat (hemiplegia) and Sandhivat as well as other Vat Janya mental diseases. Reaching the tip of the external malleolus it passes through Gulf as St41. Reaching the dorsum of the foot it forms the Kurchshir Marm as St42. Ending at the lateral side of the 2nd toe as St45. At St44 it is one of the important point for pain.

Gall-bladder Channel (Gb)—*Adhoga pittashaya dhamani* (Figure 4)

It starts from the outer canthus of the eye as Gb1 forming the Apang Marm, going horizontally as Gb2 to the posterior border of the condyloid process of mandible forming one of the point for earache.

कर्णयोरुपरि समन्तात् कर्णशूले

(सु०शा०, 8/17)

karnayorupari samantat karnashoole

(Su. Sharir, 8/17)

Then it ascends to the corner of the forehead as Gb4 and Gb14 forming the Shringatak Marm, and then curves downward reaching below occipital bone as Gb20. Reaching the hightest point of shoulder it forms ans Marm as Gb21.

Reaching directly below the free end of the 11th rib it forms Parshvasandhi Marm as Gb26. Reaching the Greater trochanter it forms important point for Gridhrasi as Gb30. Descending downward on the lateral part of the thigh at Gb31 it forms the Ani Marm. Reaching below the knee joint it forms the Janu Marm as Gb34. Reaching the Ankle joint as Gb39 it passes near to the Gulph Marm, just below it on the dorsum of foot as Gb40 it passes near to Kurchshir Marm; Ends as Gb44 at the tip of the 4th toe.

Urinary Bladder Channel (Ub)—*Adhoga mutrashaya dhamani* (Figures 17, 18, 23)

It starts from the Inner canthus of eye as Ub1(starts from Kaninika Sandhi) Ascending the forehead as Ub4 it forms the First Shringatak Marm and Ub5 as 2nd Shringatak Marm. From here it crosses the skull horizontally and posteriorly reaching Ub10 within the posterior hairline having the indication of Ansa shosh and Avabahuk. Just below in Ub11 is present as important influencing points for whole of the Skeletal system. It then bifurcates into two parts, the main channel continues to Ub41 at 3-inch lateral to 2nd thoracic vertebra along the medial aspect of the Scapula reaching Ub47, 3 inches lateral to 9th Thoracic vertebra it forms a part of Vrihati Marm. Running lateraly downward reaching Ub54, lateral to the hiatus of the sacrum it passes near to Nitamba Marm. Reaching the popliteal fossa at Ub55 with UB44 it is named as Jaldhara sira. Reaching the calf muscle at Ub58 it forms the Indra Basti Marm. Reaching laterally above the ankle joint at Ub59 it forms the Gulph Marm. At the lateral malleolus it forms the Kurch Marm as Ub61,62. Ends at Ub67 at the tip of the little toe.

Starting from Ub11 another branch runs straight downward along the medial border of Scapula over the spinous process of vertebral column reaching UB34.Many of them are the Backshu point of important organs like Lung, Heart, etc, whose roots are in the meridians and have been described by Sushrut as Srotas i.e. Pranvah Srot, Udakvah Srot etc.

Reaching Ub31 it forms Katiktarun Marm and reaching the tip of the coccyx at Ub35 it comes near gud Marm with Shukra and Artav Nadi.

Reaching the Gluteal fold it forms the Urvi Marm and ending at Ub40 in popliteal fossa it forms an important constituent of janu Marm.

TAL HRIDAYA TIRYAK DHAMANI
P: Pericardium Channel

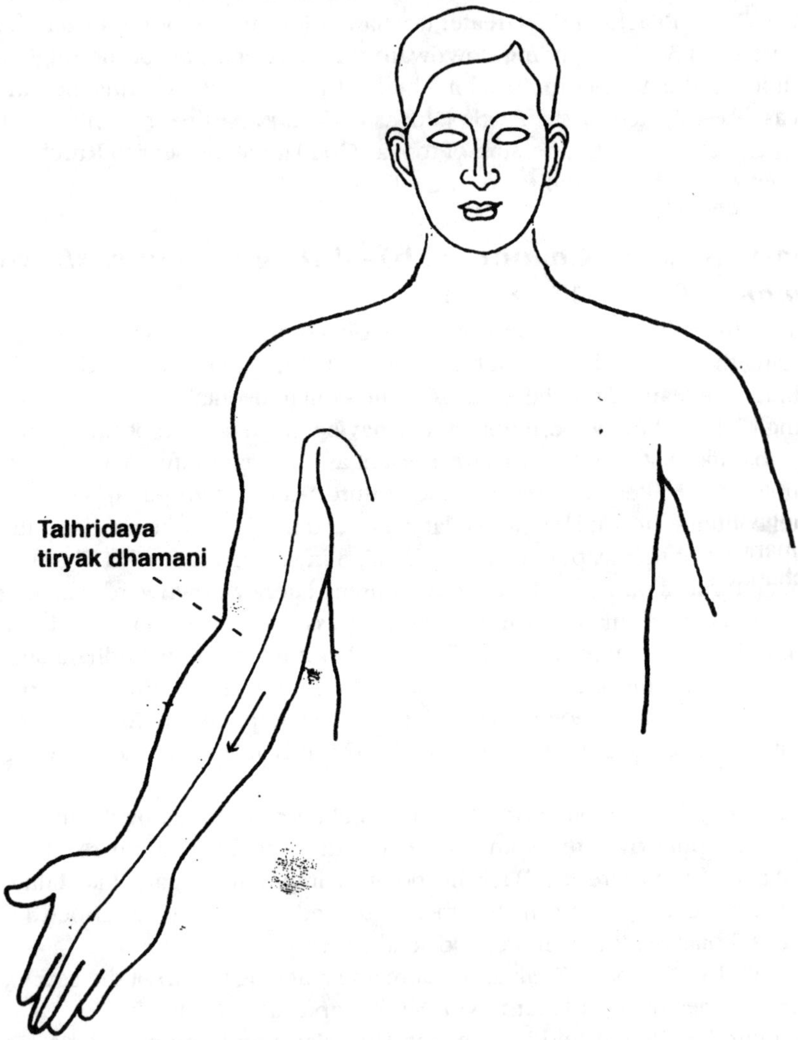

Figure 1

ADHOGA AMASHAY DHAMANI AND ADHOGA VRIHADANTRA DHAMANI

St : Stomach Channel — Li : Large Intestine Channel

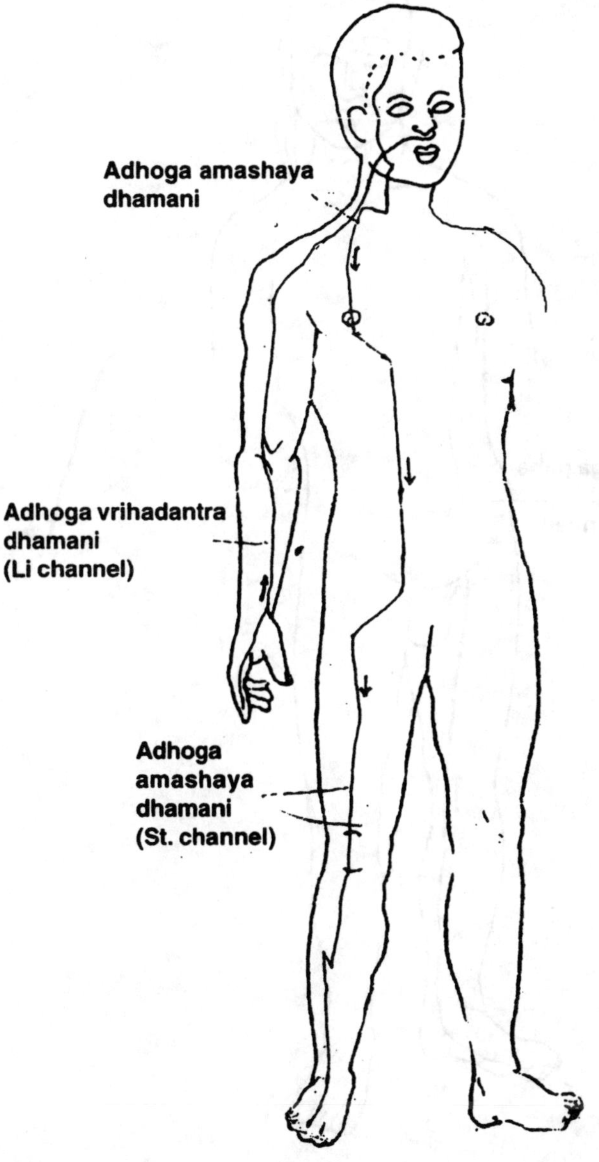

Figure 2

URDHVAGA PLIHA DHAMANI
Sp: Spleen Channel

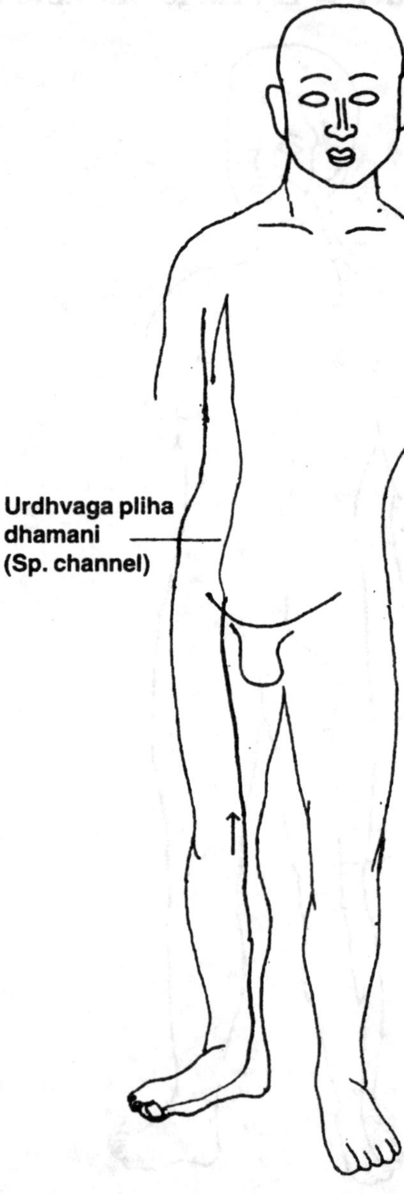

Figure 3

ADHOGA PITTASHAYA DHAMANI
Gb: Gall bladder Channel

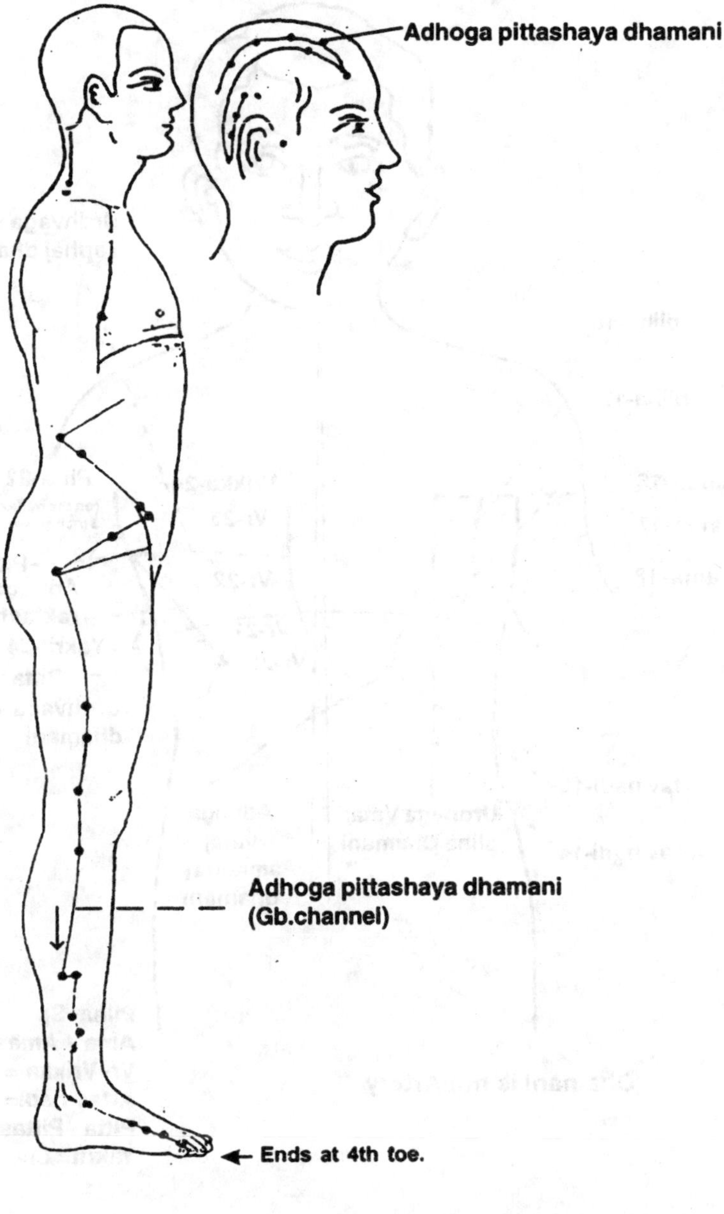

Figure 4

SIRA AND DHAMANI OF TORSO

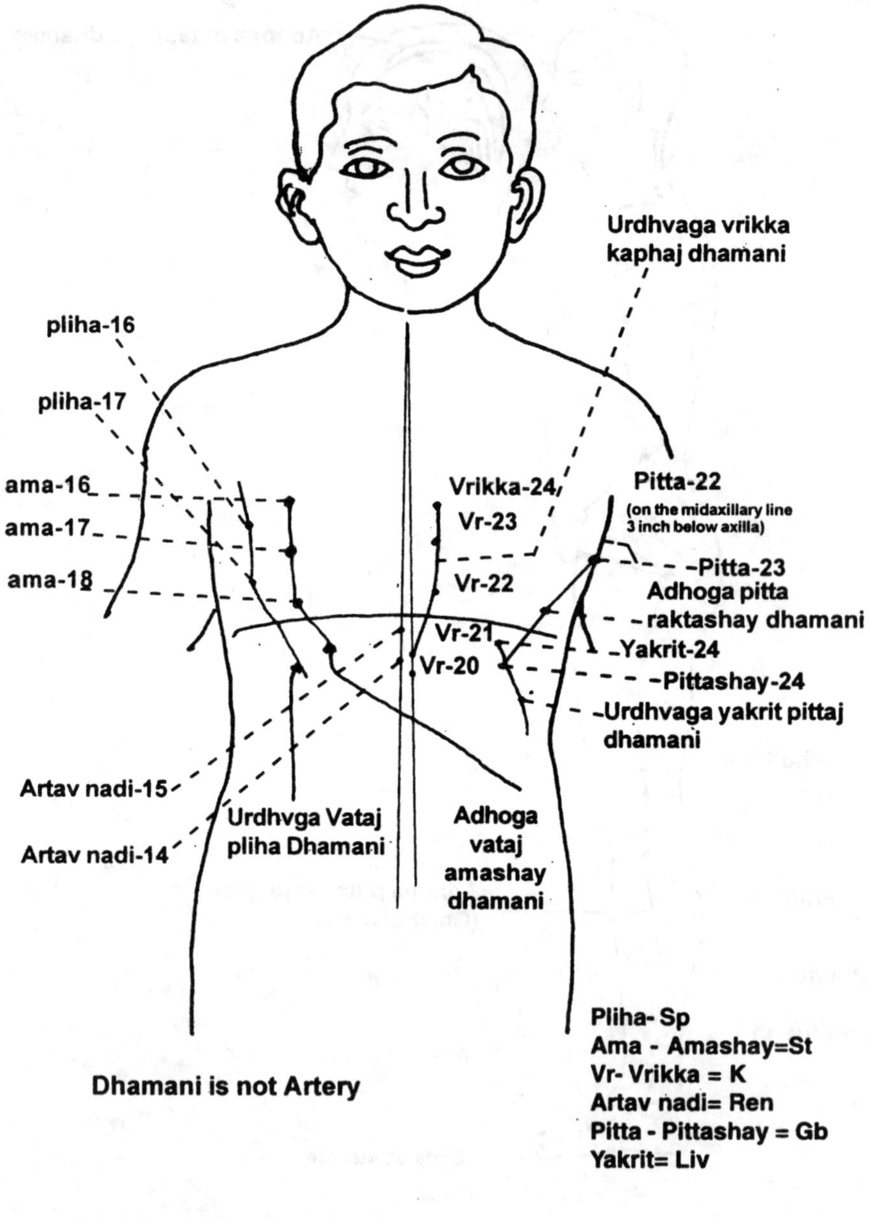

Figure 5

URDHVAGA PHUFFUS DHAMANI & VATAJ SIRA (PRANA VAYU) OF HAST (HAND)
Lung Channel (Lu)

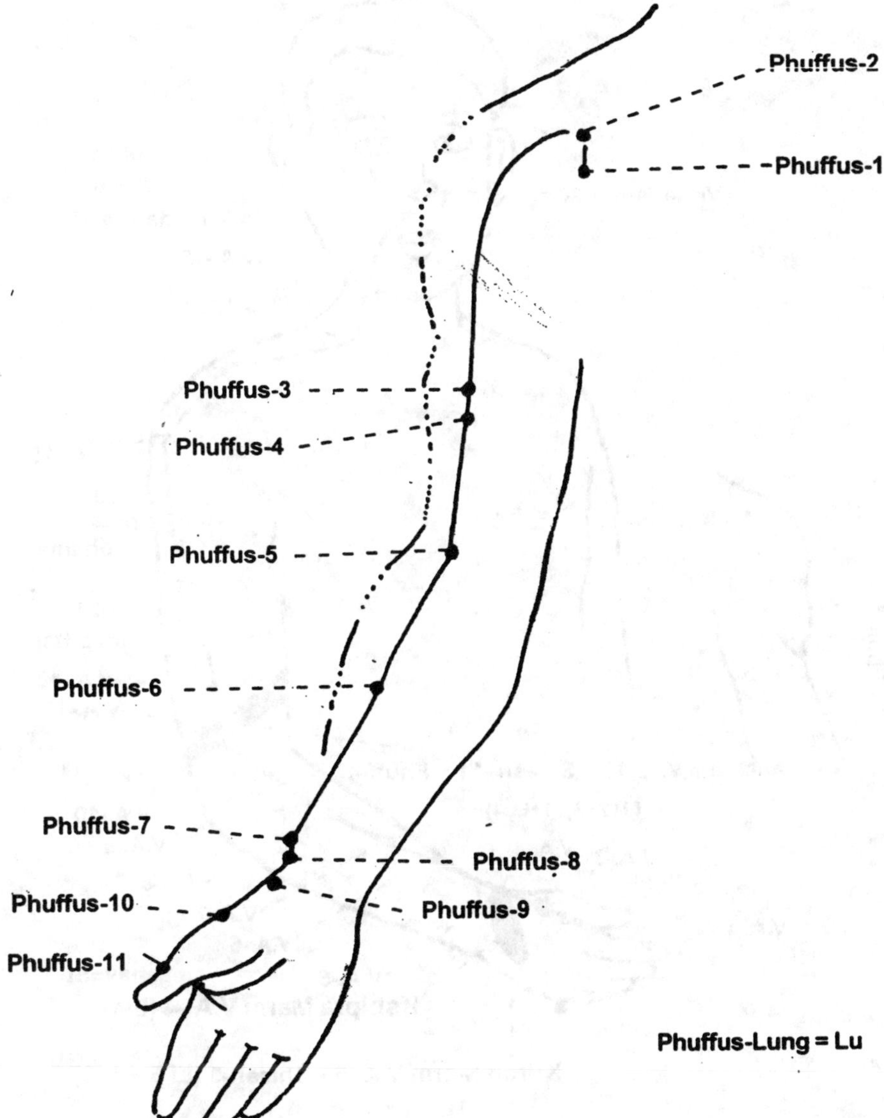

Figure 6

ADHOGA VRIHADANTRA DHAMANI (VATASHAY - APAN VAYU) & VATAJ SIRAS- PURUSH SANGYAK
LI: Large Intestine Channel - Yang

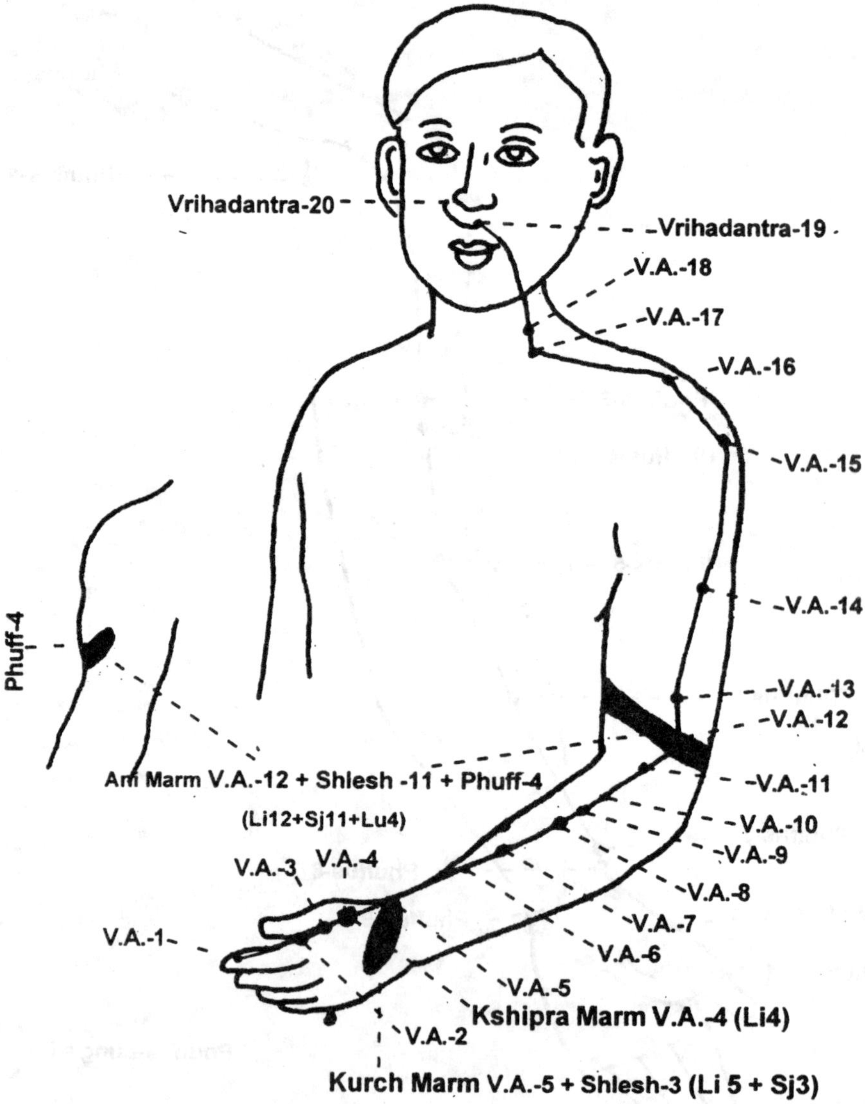

Figure 7

ADHOGA AMASHAY DHAMANI (PURUSH SANGYAK)
St - Stomach Channel Yang

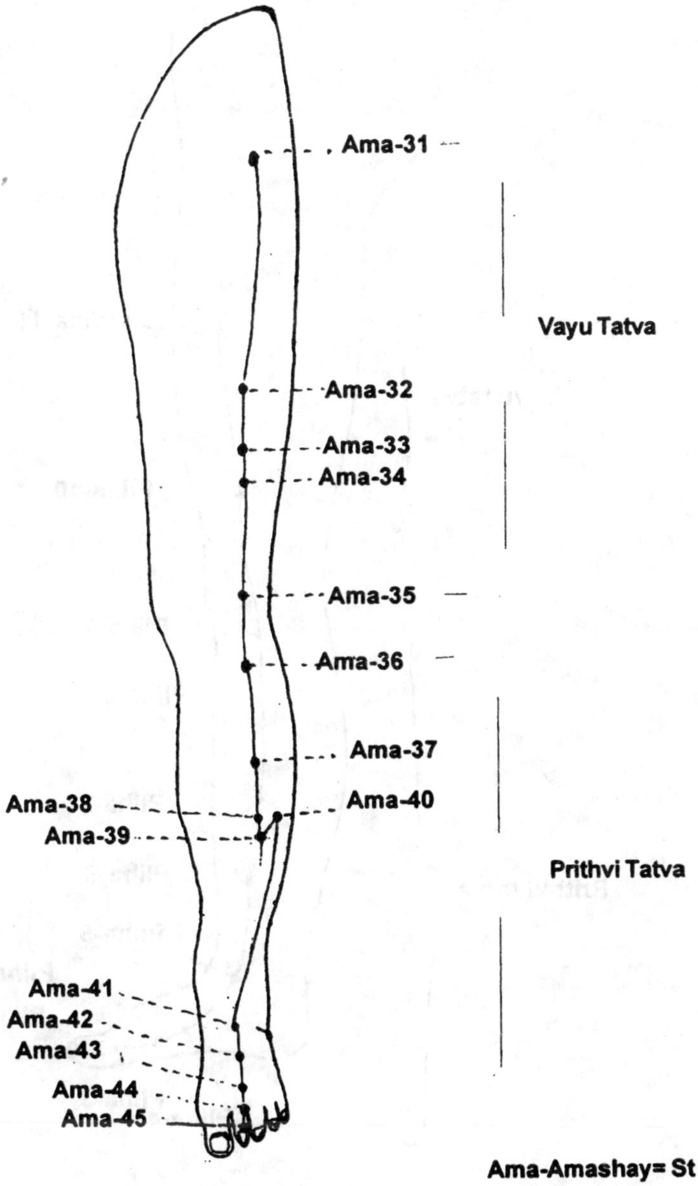

Figure 8

URDHVAGA PLIHA DHAMANI (STRI SANGYAK)
Sp: Spleen Channel (Yin)

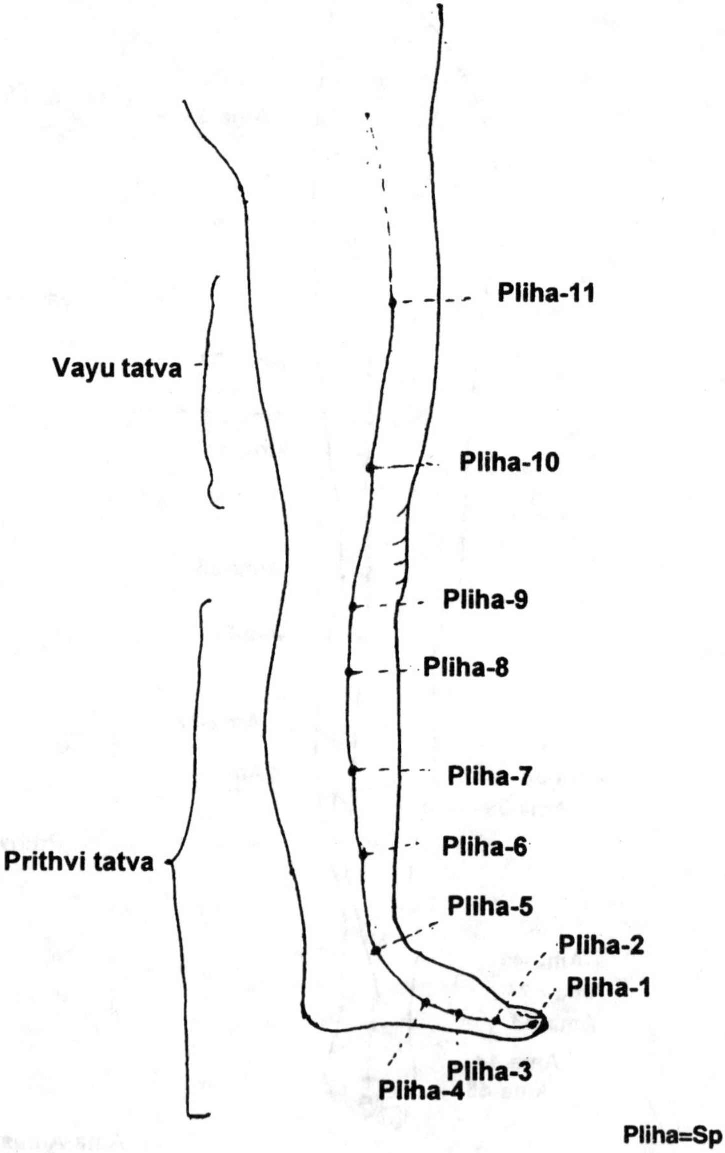

Figure 9

URDHVAGA HRIDAYA DHAMANI (DHATU PITTA & RAKTA (STRI SANGYAK) Ht (Heart Channel (Yin))

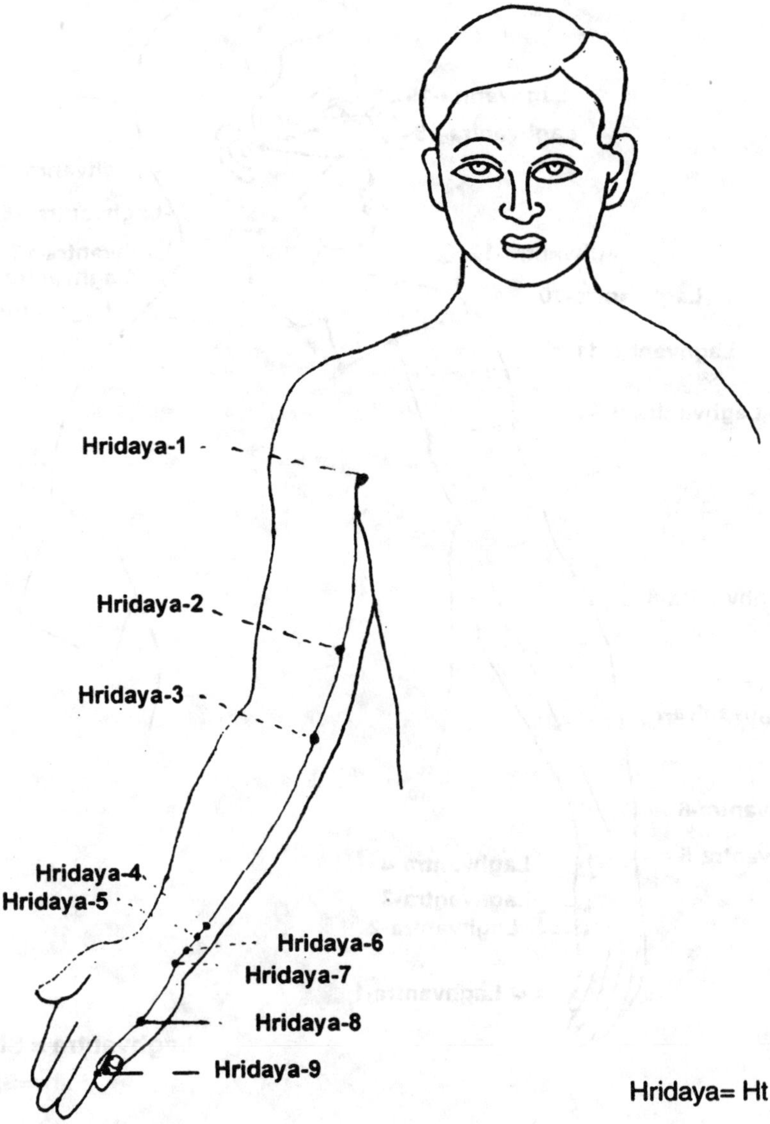

Figure 10

ADHOGA LAGHVANTRA DHAMANI & SIRA (RAKTASHAY & PITTASHAY PURUSH SANGYAK)
SI: Small Intestine channel (Yang)

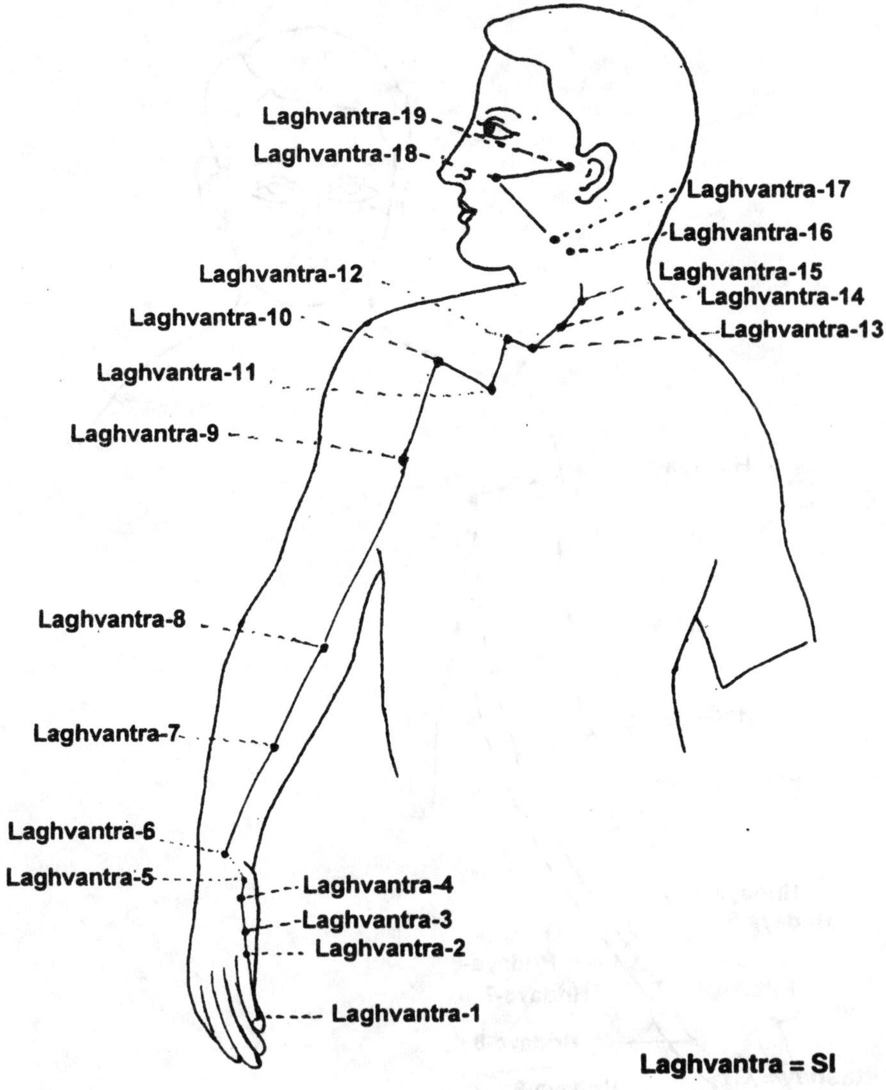

Figure 11

ADHOGA PITTASHAY DHAMANI
(Ashay - Pittashay & Raktashay - Purush Sangyak)
Gb: Gall-bladder Channel (Yang)

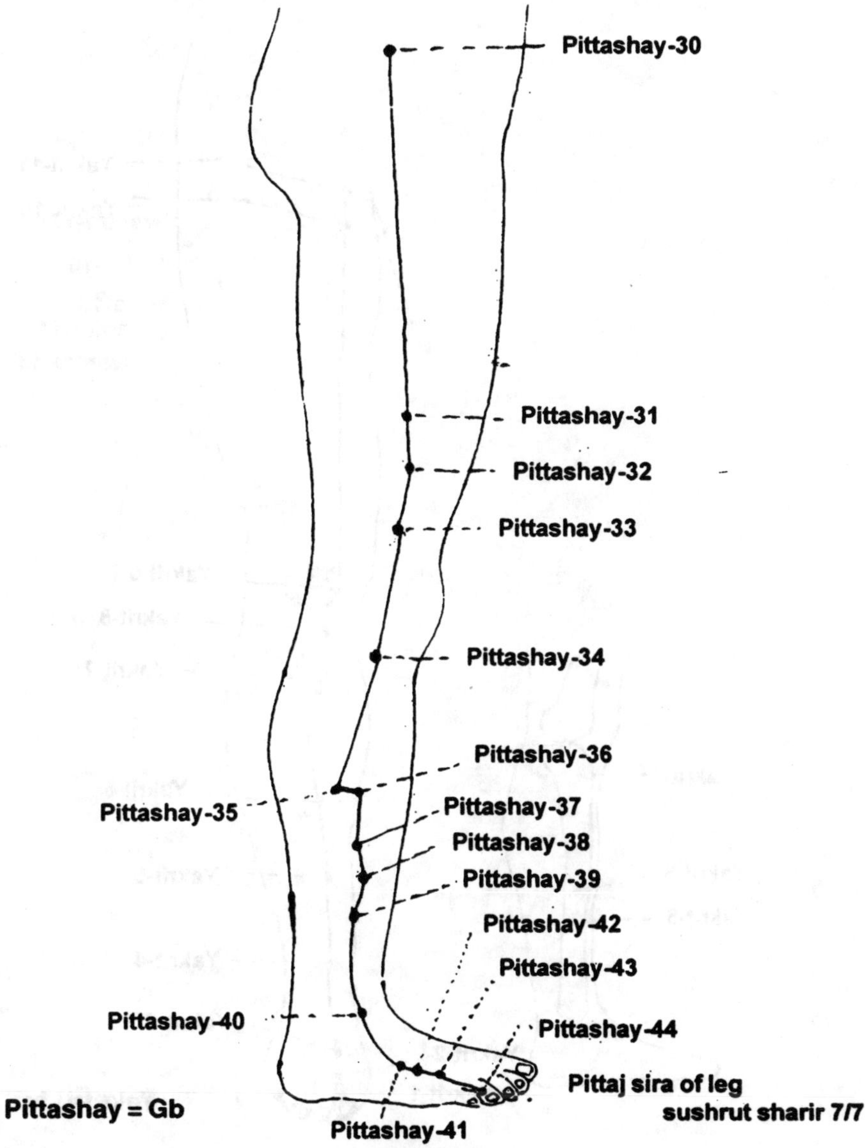

Figure 12

URDHVAGA YAKRIT DHAMANI OF PADA (LOWER EXTREMITY) (Pitta - Raktaj, Stri Sangyak) Liv: Liver Channel (Yin)

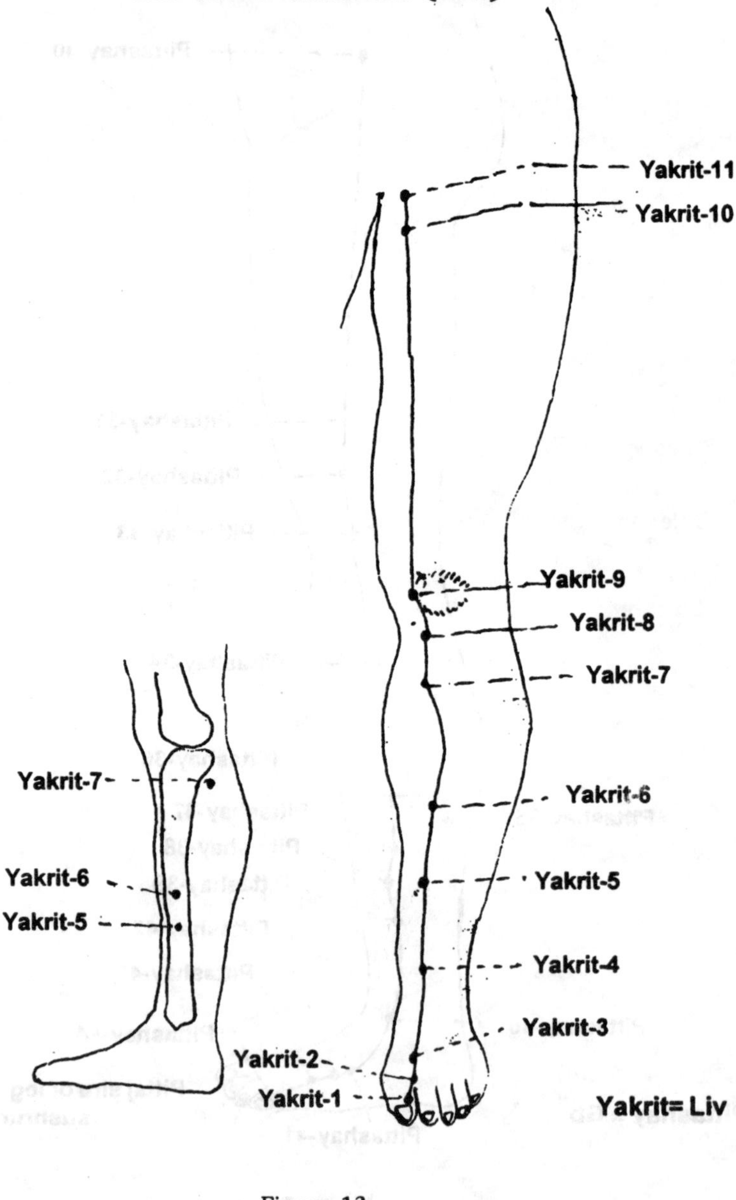

Figure 13

TIRYAGA SHLESHMASHAY DHAMANI & SIRA
(Purush Sangyak)
Sj: Sanjiao channel (Yang)

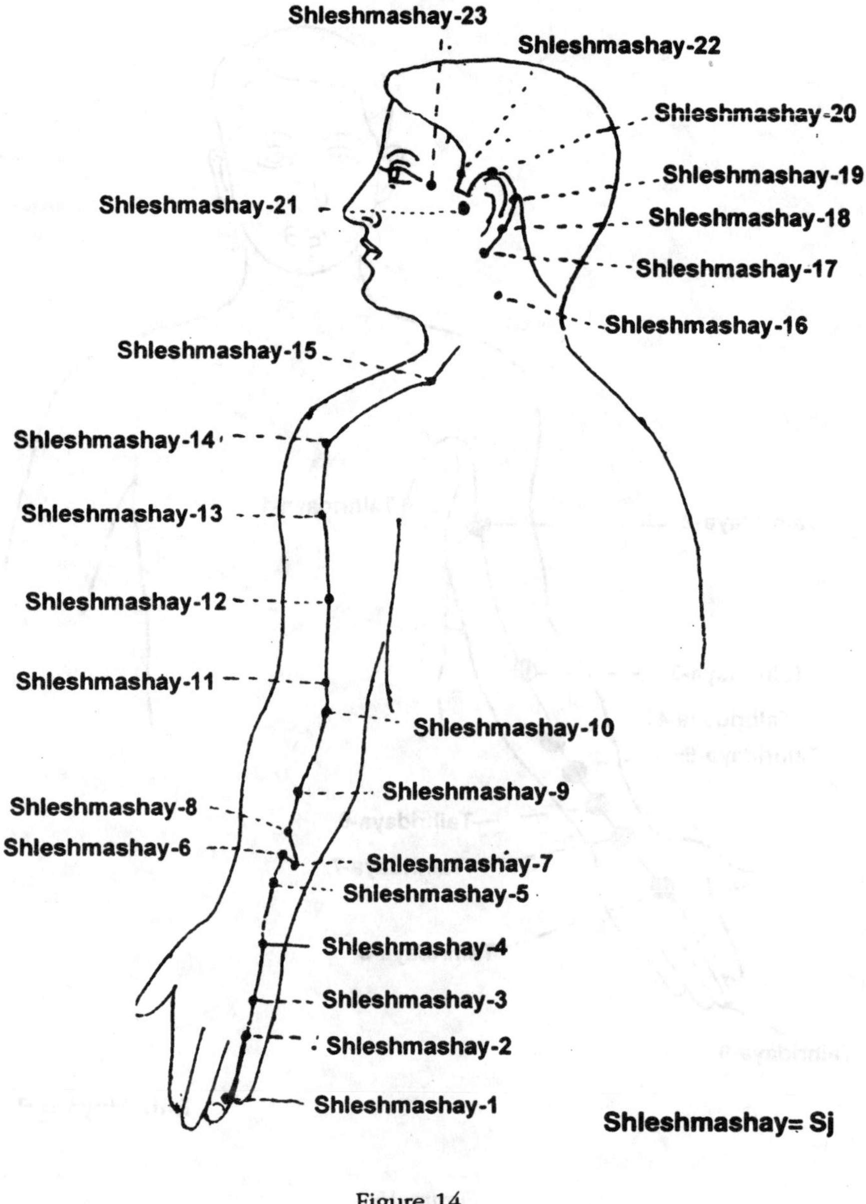

Figure 14

TIRYAGA TAL HRIDAYA DHAMANI & SIRA OF HAST (UPPER EXTREMITY) (STRI SANGYAK)
P (Pericardium Channel) Yin

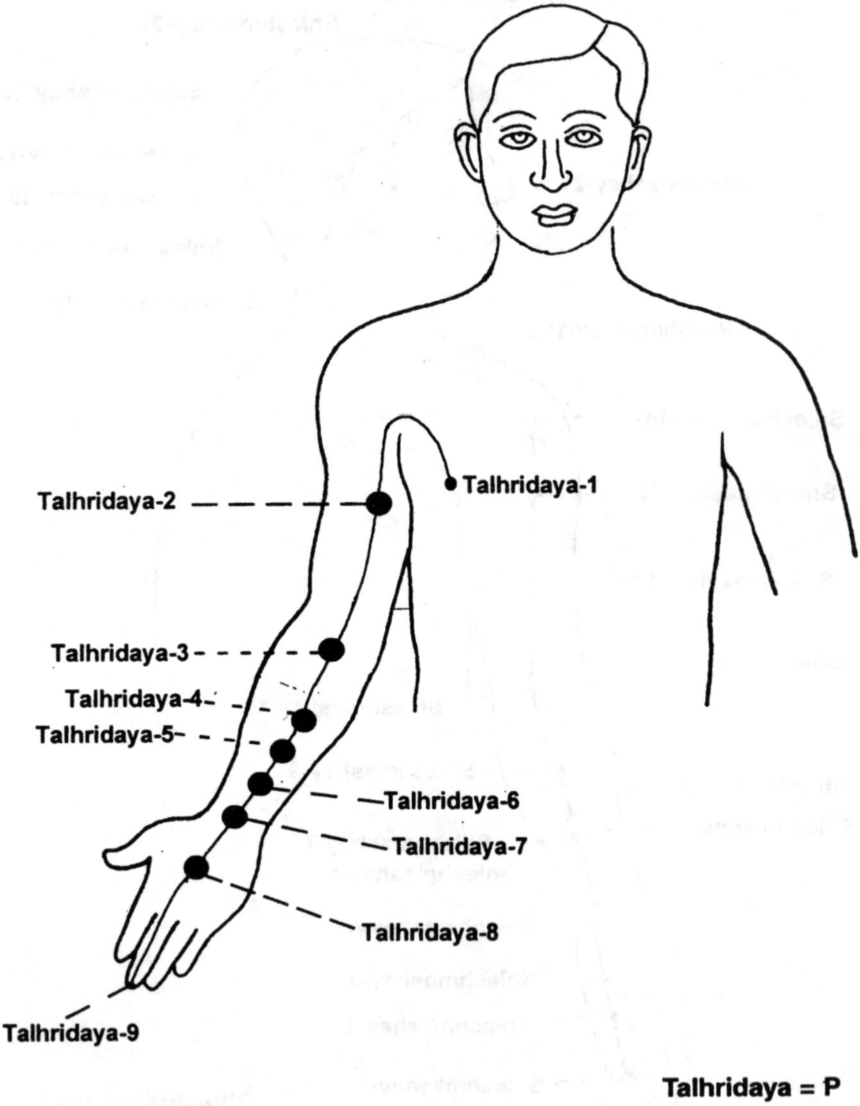

Figure 15

URDHVAGA VRIKKA DHAMANI OF SAKTHI (LOWER EXTREMITY) (KAPHAJ - STRI SANGYAK) K : Kidney Channel (Yin)

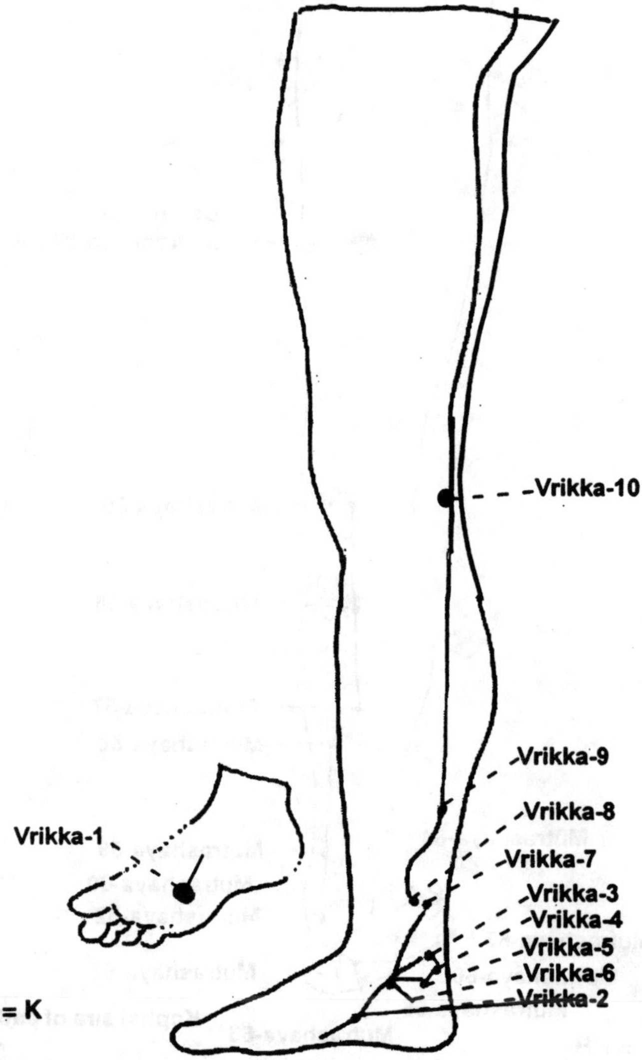

Vrikka = K

Figure 16

URVI MARM AND ADHOGA MUTRAṢHAY KAPHAJ DHAMANI (PURUSH SANGYAK)
UB: Urinary Bladder Channel (Yang)

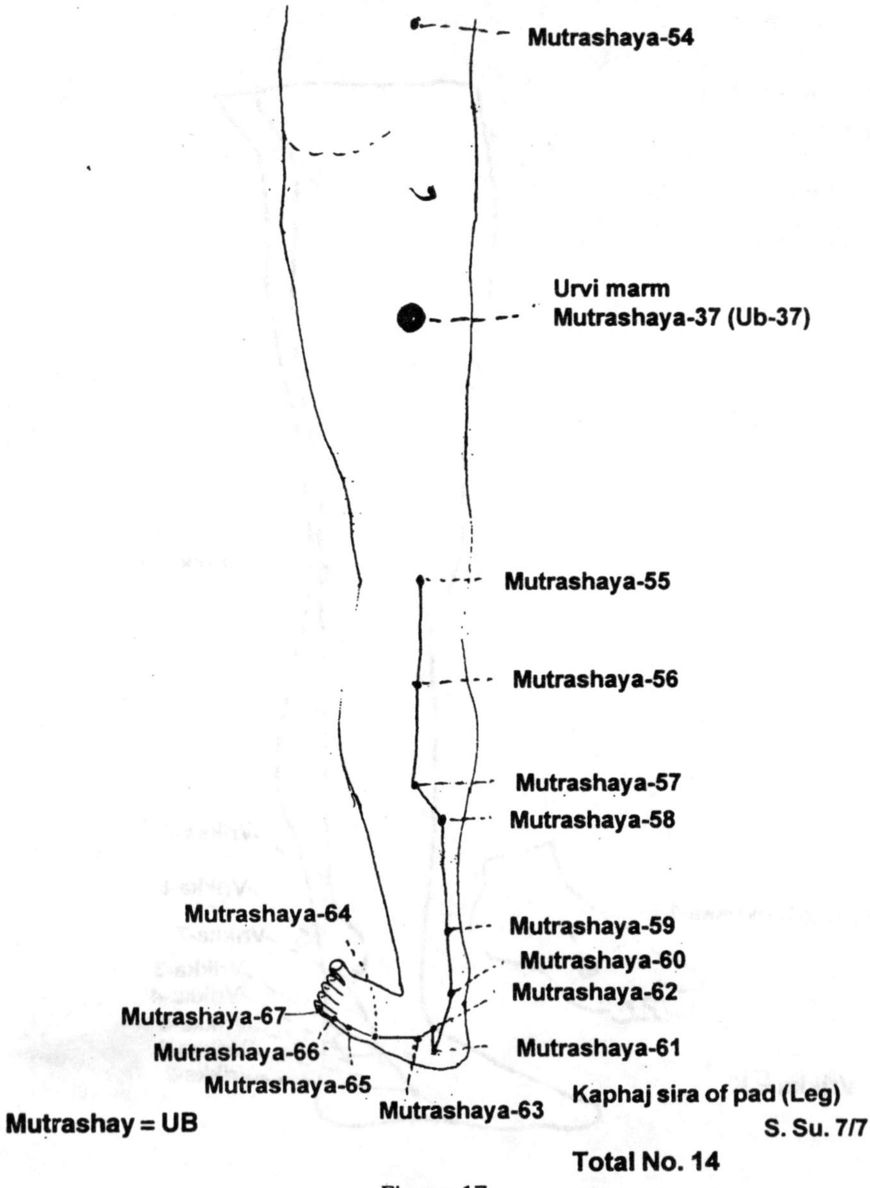

Figure 17

KAPHAJ DHAMANI AND SIRA OF URDHVAJATRU (ABOVE CLAVICLE) (UB : Urinary Bladder Channel (Mutrashay)

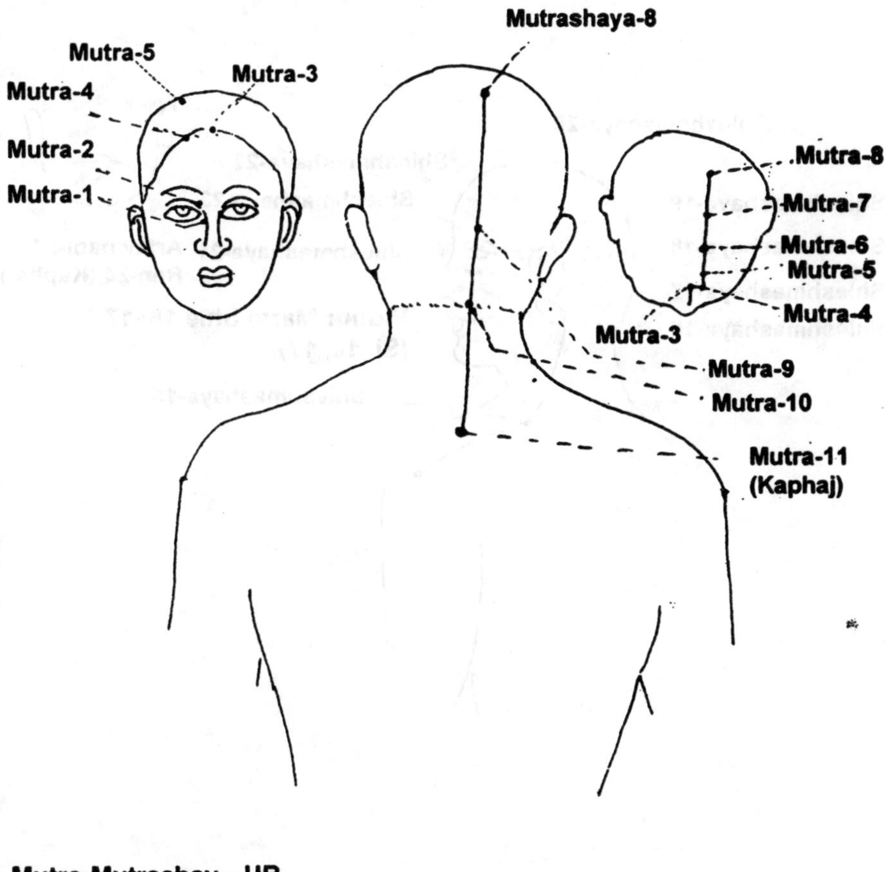

Mutra-Mutrashay = UB

Figure 18

VIDHUR MARM, KAPHAJ DHAMANI & SIRA OF URDHVAJATRU (SJ)
Sj: Sanjiao Channel.(Yang)

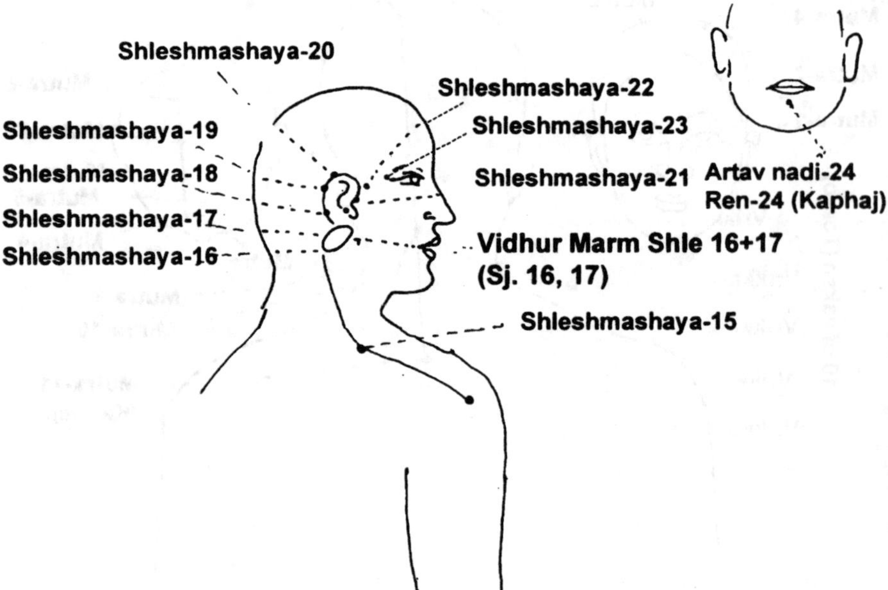

Figure 19

URDHVAGA VRIKKA DHAMANI OF KOSTH (TORSO)
K (Kidney Channel) Yin

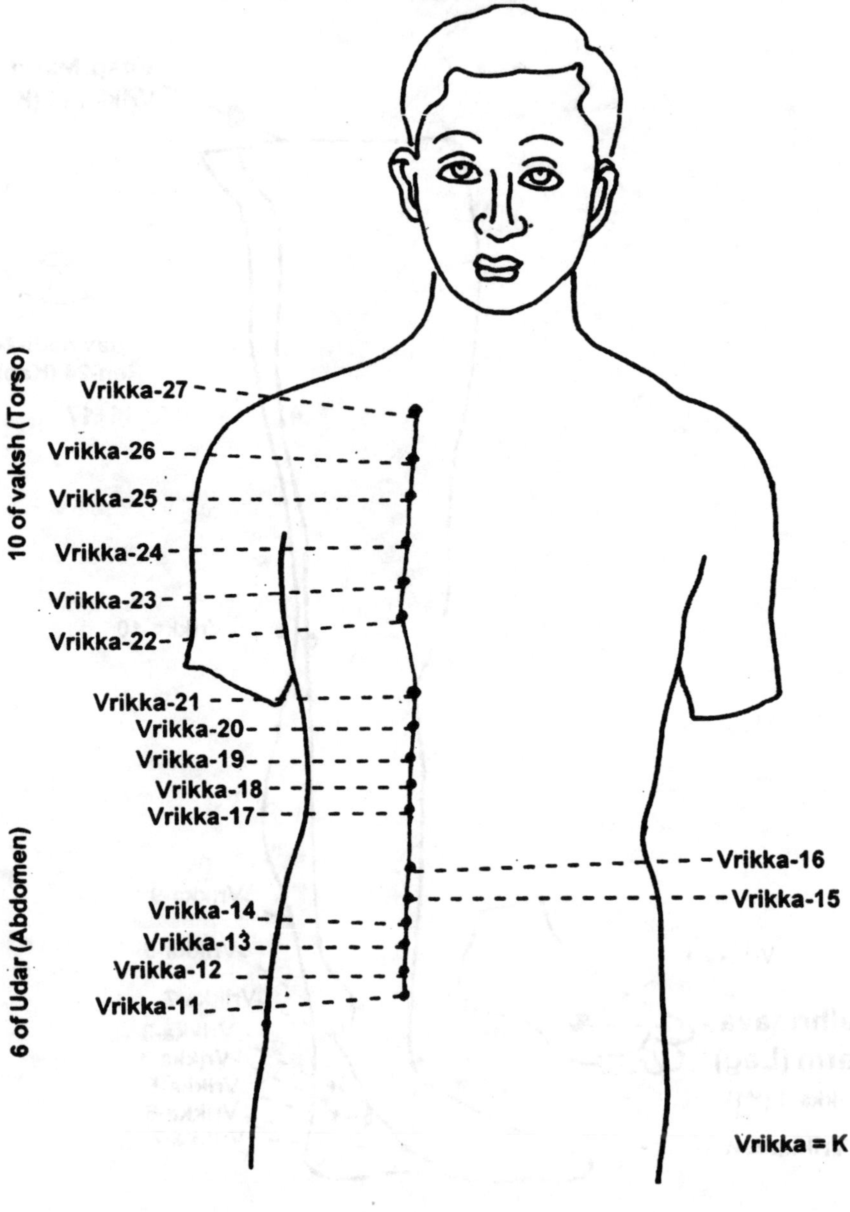

Figure 20

VRIKKA DHAMANI OF SAKTHI (LOWER EXTREMITY) (KAPHAJ - STRI SANGYAK)
K : Kidney Channel (Yin)

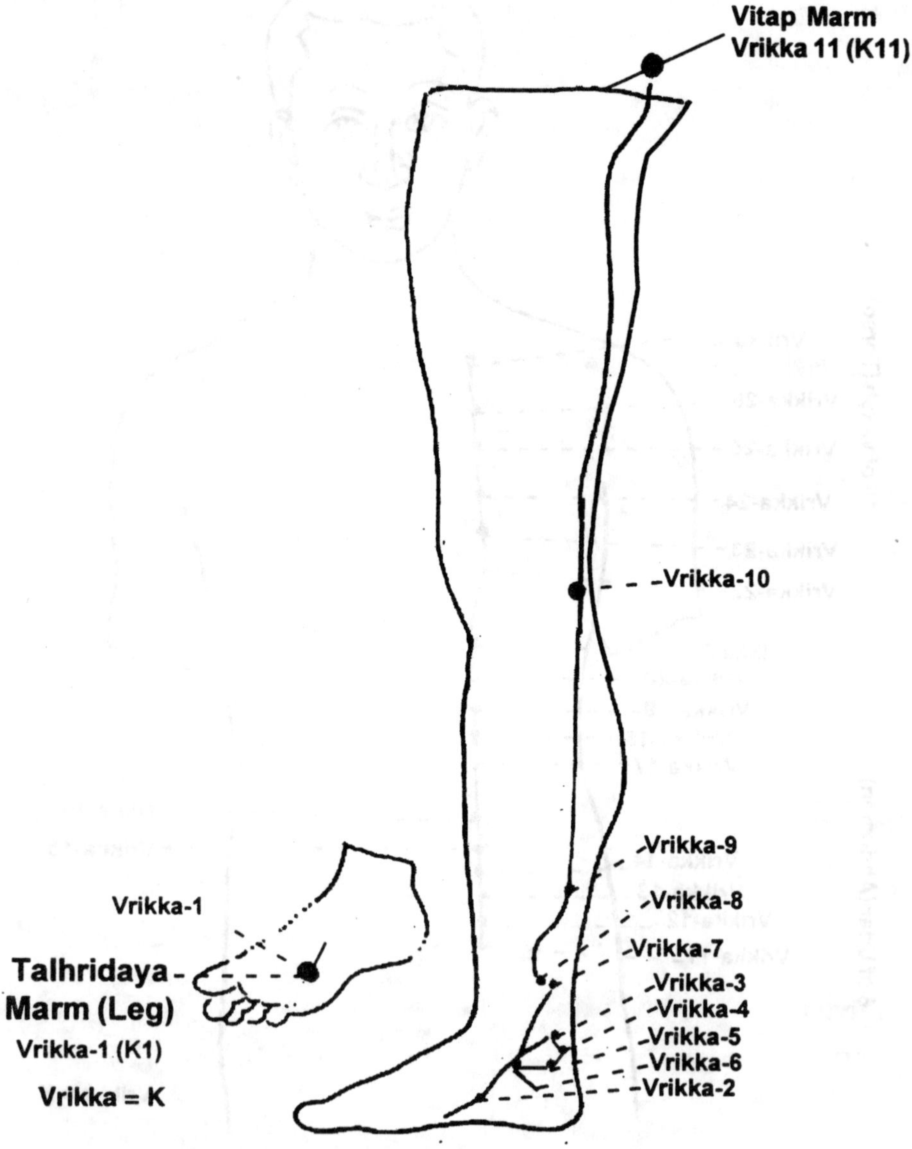

Figure 21

Chapter 3

SIRAS AND ITS DIVISION

All Dhamanis have four types of Siras embedded in their channel. Among these the original Siras are 40 in number as Sushrut says:

तासां मूलसिराश्चत्वारिंशत्; तासां वातवाहिन्यो दश, पित्तवाहिन्यो दश,कफवाहिन्यो दश, दश रक्तवाहिन्यः।
तासां तु वातवाहिनीनां वातस्थानगतानां पञ्चसप्ततिशतं भवति।

(सु०शा०, 7/6)

Tasam mulsirashçhatvarinshat; Tasam vatvahinyo dash, Pittavahinyo dash, kaphvahinyo dash, dash raktavahinyah. Tasam tu vatvahininam vatsthangatanam panchasaptatishatam bhavati ----

(Su. Sharir, 7/6)

These 40 Siras are following according to Doshas.

10 Vatvaha - Divided into 175, go to Vat-Sthan.
10 Pittavaha - Divided into 175, go to Pitta-Sthan.
10 Kaphvaha - Divided into 175, go to Kaph-Sthan.
10 Raktavaha - Divided into 175, go to Rakta-Sthan.

Raktavaha and Pittavaha have their origin in the same channel.

Siras are the points to eradicate the disease by puncturing, Agnikarm etc.

Division of 10 Vatvaha Siras of extremities (Figures 6, 7, 8, 9)

Upper extremity - Lung 1–Lu11 = 11 - Dhatu
LI 1–LI14 = 14 - Ashay
Total = 25
Lower extremity - Sp 1–Sp11 = 11 - Dhatu

	St 31–St 45	=	14 - Ashay
	Total	=	25

Note - Sirabindu St 44 & St 45 have been taken as single point because their indications are the same.
so 25 x 4 extremities = 100 Vatvaha Sira (According to Sushrut-Sharir 7/7)

Division of 10 Pittavaha Siras of Extremities (Figures 10, 11, 12, 13)

Upper extremity -	H1——H9	=	9 - Dhatu
	SI1——SI16	=	16 - Ashay
	Total	=	25
Lower extremity -	Liv1——Liv12	=	12 - Dhatu
	GB31——GB44	=	13 - Ashay
	Total	=	25

Note - Sirabindu GB43 & GB44 have been taken as single point due to their same indications.
so 25 x 4 extremities = 100 Pittavaha Siras.

Division of 10 Kaphvaha Siras of Extremities (Figures 14, 15, 16, 17)

Upper extremity -	P1——P9	=	9 - Dhatu
	Sj1——Sj16	=	16 - Ashay
	Total	=	25
Lower extremity -	K1——K11	=	11
	UB67——UB 54	=	14 - Ashay
	Total	=	25

so 25 x 4 extremities = 100 Kaphvaha Siras.

Division of 10 Raktavaha Siras of Extremities

Sushrut has counted both Pittavaha and Raktavaha Siras in the same channel because the qualities and functions of both are the same.

So the total Raktavah (as described in pittavah) are 25 x 4 = 100

So the total Siras in the extremities are 100 x 4 = 400

175 Vatvaha Sira

Total Vatvah Siras are 175 in which 100 are present in extremities and 75 are distributed in torso, head and neck. 100 siras of extremities have been already described, distribution of 75 siras of torso, head and neck are as following:

34 Vatvaha Siras of Torso

According to Sushrut Sharir 7/7, 8 Siras are located in the Shroni (Groin) under Gud (anal area) and Mehan (Penis). These are as:

Shronigat	St 30, St 29 x 2	=	4	
	Sp 12, Sp 13 x 2	=	4	
	Total	=	8	*Shronyamashtou*
Parshva (Sides)	*Dve dve parshvayo*			
	Sp 4, St 28 x 2	=	4	
Back	Du 1- Du 6	=	6	*Shat prishthe*
	(Tatra pakvashaya vishesben vat sthanam)			
Abdominal area	Sp 15, Sp 16 x 2	=	4	
	St 27 X 2	=	2	
	Total	=	6	
Chest				
	Sp 17, Sp18 x 2	=	4	
	St 18, St 17, St 16 x 2	=	6	
	Total	=	10	*Dash vakshasi*

41 Vatvaha Siras above the clavicle (Urdhvajatru) 14 in Greeva (Neck)

Ekchatvarinshajjatrunurdhva tasam chaturdash greevayam

St 13, 12, 11, 10, 9	x 2	=	10
LI 17, 18	x 2	=	4
	Total	=	14

4 in Karn (Ear) Karnayoschatastra

St 7 x 2	=	2
St 6 x 2	=	2
Total	=	4

9 in Jihva (Tongue) (Nav jihvayam) Influencing the diseases of tongue

St 9 x 2	=	2
LI 18 x 2	=	2
St 4 x 2	=	2
St 5 x 2	=	2
Du 15	=	1
Total	=	9

6 in Nasika (Nose) Shat nasikayam

LI 19 x 2	=	2
LI 20 x 2	=	2
Du 25 x 1	=	1
Du 24 x 1	=	1
Total	=	6

8 in Netra (Eyes) Ashtou netrayoh

St 1 x 2	=	2
St 2 x 2	=	2
St 8 x 2	=	2
Du 22	=	1
Du 23	=	1
Total	=	8

So total 75 +100 Siras of extremities = 175 Vatvah Siras.

175 Pittavaha Siras

Total Pittavaha Siras are 175 in which 100 are present in extremities and 75 are distributed in torso, head & neck. 100 Siras of extremities have been already described, Distribution of 75 Siras of torso, head & neck are as follows:

34 Pittavaha Siras in kosth (Torso)

8 in Shroni (Groins) over the Gud (Anal area) & Mehan (Penis)

GB 28 x 2	=	2
GB 27 x 2	=	2
Ren 7 x 1	=	1

Note - Remaining 3 Pittavaha Siras of Sroni could not be determined and located.

2 on the Parshva (each side)

Liv 13 X 2	=	2
GB 25 X 2	=	2
	=	4

6 on the Back (Prishtha)

GB 25 X 2	=	2
GB 30 X 2	=	2
GB 29 X 2	=	2
		6

6 in Abdominal area (udar)

Ren1 - 6	=	6

Ren 4 is Front Mu Point of Small intestine hence it is pittaj sira

10 over the Chest (Vaksha-Sthal)

Liv 14 x 2	=	2
GB 22 x 2	=	2
GB 23 x 2	=	2
GB 24 x 2	=	2
Ren 14	=	1

Ren 15 = 1 Front Mu point of heart so it is Pittaj sira

41 Pittavahini Sira above the clavicle (Urdhva Jatru) 14 in neck (Greeva)

Ekchatvarinshajjatrunurdhva tasam chaturdash greevayam

GB 21 x 2	=	2
GB 20 x 2	=	2
SI 17 x 2	=	2
SI 16 x 2	=	2
SI 15 x 2	=	2
SI 14 x 2	=	2
SI 13 x 2	=	2

2 going in to Ears

SI 19 x 2	=	2

10 going in to the eyes

GB 1 X 2	=	2
GB 4 X 2	=	2
GB 5 X 2	=	2
GB 13 X 2	=	2
GB 14 X 2	=	2

9 going into the tongue

Ren 23	=	1
SI 18 x 2	=	2
GB 2 x 2	=	2
GB 3 x 2	=	2
GB 7 x 2	=	2

6 affecting nose

GB 18 x 2	=	2
GB 15 x 2	=	2
GB 20 x 2	=	2

175 Kaphaj Siras

According to Sushrut,total number of Kaphaj Siras are 175. Their distribution are as follows:

Shakha (Extremities)	-	100
Koshth (Torso)	-	34
Urdhvajatru (Above clavicle)	-	41

Distribution of 100 Kaphaj Siras of Extremities (Figures 14, 15, 16, 17)

Upper extremities

P1 - 9	=	9
Sj1 - 16	=	16
25 x 2	=	50

Lower extremities

K1 – 11	=	11
UB 67 – 54	=	14
25 X 2	=	50

Distribution of 34 Kaphaj Siras of Torso: (Figure 17, 20, 36)

8 in Groin (Shroni) affecting Anus (Gud) and Penis (Mehan)

K 12, 13, 14, 15 x 2 = 8

2 each on each side of the Groin (Figure 20)

K 25, 26 x 2 = 4

6 in Back (Prishtha)

UB 47, UB 53, UB54 x 2 = 6

6 in Abdomen (udar) (Figure 20)

K 17, 18, 19 x 2 = 6

10 in chest (Figure 20)

K 20, 21, 22, 23, 24 X 2 = 10

41 Kaphaj Siras above the clavicle (Urdhvajatru) (Figures 18,19)

UB 1 - 11 x 2	=	22
SJ 15 - 23 x 2	=	18
Ren 24	=	1
		41

175 Raktavaha Siras:

Because of identical qualities, properties and causes of vitiation, Sushrut has counted Raktavaha and Pittavaha Siras in same channel.

अनुष्णशीतं मधुरं स्निग्धं रक्तं च वर्णतः।
शोणितं गुरु विस्रं स्याद्विदाहश्चास्य पित्तवत् ।।

(सु०सू०, 21/17)

Anushnashitam madhuram snigdham raktam ch varntah
Shonitam guru visram syadvidahashchasya pittavat

(Sushrut Sutra, 21/17)

शोणितस्य स्थानं यकृत्प्लीहानौ

(सु०सू०, 21/16)

Shonitasya sthanam yakritpleehanou

(Sushrut Sutra, 21/16)

यत्तु यकृत्प्लीह्नोः पित्तं तस्मिन्
रञ्जकोऽग्निरिति संज्ञा।

(सु०सू०, 21/10)

Yattu yakritpleehnoh pittam tasmin ranjakoagniriti sangya

(Sushrut Sutra, 21/10)

The causes of vitiation of Raktadhatu and Pittadhatu are the same

पित्तप्रकोपेणैरेव चाभीक्ष्णं -------------

(सु०सू०, 21/25)

Pittaprakopanairev chabhikshnam ....

(Sushrut Sutra, 21/25)

Chapter 4

AVEDHYA SIRAS AND SIRAVYADH VIDHI

Avedhya Siras—The Siras where Siravedhan (needling) is contra-indicated

Needling is contraindicated in the following Siras or points:

16 Siras in the extremities
32 Siras in the torso (Koshth)
50 Siras in the head (Shir)

Please consult *Sushrut Sharir-Sthan,* 7/22, for their location and further detail.

In emergencies, however, when life is at stake, needling can be performed only by expert hand who have full command of Anatomy without puncturing and damaging the main arteries, plexuses and vital delicate structures.

Siravyadh Vidhi—Technique of Siravedhan (Acupuncture)

The therapeutic acupuncture is performed to promote smooth circulation of Ras (Prana) and blood.

According to *Sushrut Sharir,* 8/7, Siravyadhan (Therapeutic Acupuncture) should not be performed under following conditions:

नैवातिशीते नात्युष्णे न प्रवाते न चाभ्रिते।
सिराणां व्यधनं कार्यमरोगे वा कदाचन।।

(सु० शा०, 8/7)

Naivatishite natyushne na pravate na chabhrite,
Siranam vyadhanam karyamroge va kadachan .

(Sushrut Sharir, 8/7)

Siravyadhan (Acupuncture) should not be performed in very cold weather, very hot weather, during storm, during cloudy days and without any indication. Acharya Sushrut has specifically stressed upon the correct timings of procedure, selection of proper site for the procedure, selection of instruments and their sterilization must be done before hand (See *Sushrut Sutra 5/7*).

According to Sushrut following should be the qualities of therapist:

शौर्यमाशुक्रिया शस्त्रतैक्ष्णयमस्वेदवेपथू।
असम्मोहश्च वैद्यस्य शस्त्रकर्मणि शस्यते।।

(सु०सू०, 5/10)

Shoryamashukriya shastrataikshanyamasvedvepathu,
Asammohashch vaidhyasya shastrakarmani shasyate.

(Sushrut Sutra, 5/10)

The therapist should be courageous, fast and having sharp instruments. He should neither be afraid nor worried of work and he should perform his work with deliberateness.

In Sushrut Sutra 5/122, Acharya has allowed more than one puncture. If therapeutic result is not seen by single puncture then more than one puncture should be done. Oblique insertion of the needle should be performed in the following areas:

तत्र भ्रूगण्डशङ्खललाटाक्षिपुठौष्ठदन्तवेष्टकक्षाकुक्षि
वङ्क्षणेषु तिर्यक् छेद उक्तः।

(सु०सू०, 5/13)

Tatra bhrugandashankh lalatakshiputhoshth dantveshta
Kaksha kukshi vangshaneshu tiryak ched uktah

(Sushrut Sutra, 5/13)

Sushrut indicates oblique insertion in Bhru (Eyebrow), Gandsthal (Side of the face and neck), Shankhpradesh (Temple), Lalat (fore head), Akshivartm (Eyelids), Kaksha(Axilla), Kukshi(Abdomen),Vankshan(Groins).

Further, straight insertion should be performed in the sole and palm. Semicircular over anal area and penis perpendicular in rest of the places. (*Sushrut Sutra, 5/14*)

In Sushrut Sharir-8 Acharya Sushrut has described different postures of the patient for different diseases as in Sciatica and frozen shoulder, the Knee joint and elbow should be fully flexed respectively.

Depth of Needle (See *Sushrut Sharir,* 8/9)

In muscular areas the depth of puncturing should be yav - matra (5mm). For other places or for areas above the bones the depth should be 2.5mm *(Ardh yav)* and the instrument should be broad edged as *Kutharika Shastra.* According to Shusrut Sharir 8/11 proper puncture immediately stops pain by initiating the flow of blood. According to Sushrut Sharir 8/14, in weak persons puncturing should be repeated not earlier than 2 or 3 days.

In Sushrut Sharir 8/22-23, Sushrut emphasises the importance of Siravedhan (acupuncture):

स्नेहादिभिः क्रियायोगैर्न तथा लेपनैरपि।
यान्त्याशु व्याधयः शान्तिं यथा सम्यक् सिराव्यधात्।।
सिराव्यधश्चिकित्सार्धं शल्यतन्त्रे प्रकीर्तितः।

(सु०शा०, 8/22-23)

Snehadibhih kriyayogairn tatha lepnairapi
Yantyashu vyadhayah shantim yatha samyak siravyadhat
Siravyadhashchikitsardham shalyatantre prakertitah

(Sushrut Sharir, 8/22–23)

The medicines, ointments are not as effective and rapid in action as acupuncture is.

By saying *'Shiravyadhashchikitsardham'* Sushrut says that Siravedh (acupuncture) procedure is half of the other treatment procedures.

Chapter 5

SROT

According to *Sushrut Sharir*, 9/13 Srot are not situated in regular channels like regular Dhamani (Channels) and Siras (points above dhamanis). These are somewhat more important and are directly related with the main organ:

मूलात् खादन्तरं देहे प्रसृतं त्वभिवाहि यत् ।

(सु०शा० 9/13)

Moolat khadantaram dehe prasritam tvabhivahi yat

(Sushrut Sharir, 9/13)

According to *Sushrut Sharir 9/12*, the total number of Srot are 22.

1.	Pranvah Srot	—	2
2.	Annavah Srot	—	2
3.	Udakvah Srot	—	2
4.	Rasvah Srot	—	2
5.	Raktavah Srot	—	2
6.	Mansvah Srot	—	2
7.	Medvah Srot	—	2
8.	Mutravah Srot	—	2
9.	Purishvah Srot	—	2
10.	Shukravah Srot	—	2
11.	Artavvah Srot	—	2

In *Sushrut Sharir*, 9/12, he says that when the srot (mool) of these Srot get diseased or afflicted the symptoms occurs according to the related organ. As for example when heart (related with Pranvah Srot) gets diseased the symptoms will be shouting in anger, bending with shooting pain in heart, fainting, giddiness, tremors and ultimately death and the cure of this ailment of heart is long-term stimulation of its Pranavah Srot UB15 by needle or Agnikarm.

The stimulation points [*Srotas* (mukh)—holes] are present in the urinary bladder channels of back (*Prishtha*). These UB points from UB12 to UB40 are not counted in regular channels (dhamani or siras) but Sushrut counted them under the heading of Srot:

Name	*Mukh*	*Related organ*
1. Pranvah Srot	UB15	Heart (Hridaya, H)
2. Annavah Srot	UB21	Stomach(Amashay, St.)
3. Udakvah Srot	UB20	Spleen (Pliha, Sp.)
4. Rasvah Srot	UB14	Pericardium (Talhridaya, P)
5. Raktavah Srot	UB18	Liver (Yakrit, Liv.)
6. Mansvah Srot	UB13	Lung (Phuffus, Lu)
7. Medvah Srot	UB 23	Kidney (Vrikka, K)
8. Mutravah Srot	UB 28	Urinary Bladder (Mutrashay, Ub)
9. Purishvah Srot	UB 25	Large Intestine (Vrihdantra, Li)
10. Shukravah Srot	UB 22	Sanjiao (Shleshmashay, Sj)
11. Artavvah Srot	UB 27	Small Intestine (Laghvantra, Si)

We determined UB19, mukh of Gall-bladder as Raktavaha Srot again, to complete the Mukh or to treat the complete 24 channels.

In Sushrut Sharir 9/12, Sushrut says that when these Srotas get diseased or afflicted its treatment is long term stimulation. *(Srotoviddham tu pratyakhyeyopcharet—Su.Sh., 9/12)*.

So one should perform long-term stimulation of these UB Point (Mukh) with the help of Siravedh (needling) or Agnikarm.

Chapter 6

MARM

According to *Sushrut Sharir-Sthan-6,* the therapeutic puncturing points (Marmas) are 107 in number. Marmas are of five types—Mans Marm, Sira Marm,Snayu Marm, Asthi Marm and Sandhi Marm. The vital energies (Pran) are locked up in these marmas, therefore, when they are damaged by disease, the power of sense of vital organs like eyes, ears; heart, lungs, kidneys is also affected.

The innerconscious—'self' has the wisdom to operate that selfcure mechanism. It comes into operation only when the indicated Sira or Marm is activated by Acupuncture (Siravedh), Moxibustion (Agni Karm), Kshar or application of Leeches (Su.Sutra 13/4). Sushrut has appreciated Kshar as Tridosh-Nashak. (Sushrut Sutra 11/13).

Sushrut has recommended Agnikarm (Moxibustion)for many selective diseases. He has described four stages of Agni Karm as Plushta, Durdagdha, Samyag dagdha and Atidagdha (Su.Sutra 12/16). He has also described the selective types of Agnikarm as Valaya, Bindu, Vilekha etc. For blood letting he has recommended Leeches as best for Paittik as well as Raktaj diseases (Su.Sutra 13/4). The previously mentioned Siras are situated in Marmas (see Su.Sha 6/18). Sushrut has used the term 'Marm' both for diseases of vital organ-system as well as the topographical cure points, therefore the Marm in the system should be saved by stimulating topographical cure points (Sushrut Sharir 6/33).

The Marmas also have another prophylactic use against several ailments as in well as conferring immunity and enhancing resistance against diseases. For this purpose mild stimulation for three to four days is required. In those cases where Sushrut has described immediate fatal instances (Sadya-Pranhar Marm) e.g. in Hridaya Marm-prophylactic acupuncture or stimulation should be performed. These are called alarm points which can check the impending attack. These are athletes vitality and revival points also. These are the points mentioned in the Yajurvedic System of Medicine as Mahamrityunjay Mantra (Victory over death).

The word Aghat or Abhighat, used by Sushrut, means the loss of vitality power i.e. in Abhighat of Kshipra-Marm, the blood coagulation power decreases, the whole blood coagulating system gets disturbed i.e., Vitamin K, Coagulation factor, fibrinogens etc. disappear and consequently death occurs due to haemorrhages of any organ (see *Su.Sh.*, 6/32). It is a wrong interpretation that due to Aghat of Kshipra Marm bleeding will occur from its points Li 4 or Liv 3.

Number of Marmas

Mans Marm	Sira Marm	Snayu Marm	Asthi Marm	Sandhi Marm
11	41	27	8	20

Topography of the Marmas

Lower Extremity	11 x 2 = 22
Upper Extremity	11 x 2 = 22
Abdomen and Chest	12
Back	14
Above Clavicle	37

Nomenclature of Marmas

Lower Extremity:

Kshipra
Talhridaya
Kurcha
Kurchashir
Gulpha
Indravasti
Janu
Ani
Urvi
Lohitaksha
Vitap

Upper Extremities

Kshipra
Talhridaya
Kurcha
Kurchashir
Manibandh
Lohitaksha
Indravasti
Kurpar
Ani
Urvi
Kakshadhar

Abdomen and Chest

Guda	Stanmool
Vasti	Stanrohit
Nabhi	Apalap
Hridaya	Apastambh

Back

Katiktarun	Vrihati
Kukundar	Ansaphalak
Nitamba	Ans
Parshva Sandhi	

Above Clavicle

Dhamanis	- 4	Avart	- 2
Matrika	- 8	Utkshep	- 2
Krikatika	- 2	Shankh	- 2
Vidhur	- 2	Sthapni	- 1
Fan	- 2	Simant	- 5
Apang	- 2	Shringatak	- 4 and Adhipati - 1

Mansmarm

All Mans Marmas are in yin plane (Urdhvaga) on fleshy portion of the body:

Talhridaya	Guda
Indravasti	Stanrohit

Sira Marm

The Sira Marms are generally located near important arteries, veins and plexuses:

Neel dhamani	Apalap
Matrika	Apastambha
Shringatak	Hridaya
Apang	Nabhi
Sthapni	Parshvasandhi
Fan	Brihati
Stanmool	Lohitaksha
Urvi	

Snayu Marma

By Snayu we mean braincells, motor and sensory neurons, central cortex, nerves, tendons and whole of the nervous system and following Marmas come under it:

Ani	Vasti
Vitap	Kshipra
Kakshadhar	Ans
Kurch	Vidhur
Kurchshir	Utkshep

Asthi Marm

All these marmas lie above the bony portion:

Katiktarun	Ansaphalak
Nitamba	Shankh

Sandhi Marm

These Marmas are placed over the important joints of the body:

Janu	Manibandh
Kurpar	Kukundar
Simant	Avart
Adhipati	Krikatika
Gulph	

Classification of Marmas according to their fatality and pain Syndromes

Sadhya Pranhar (instant death) Marmas:

Following marmas are called Sadhya Pranhar because the death occurs due to shock and vasovagal attack.

Shringatak	Guda
Adhipati	Hridaya
Shankh	Vasti
Kanthsira	Nabhi

Kalantar Pranhar Marmas:

Kalantar Pranhar Marmas are the Marmas where prognosis is bad due to uncontrolled haemorrhage.

All Vaksha Marmas (Marmas in Chest)	Katiktarun
Simant	Parshvasandhi
Talhridaya	Brihati
Kshipra	Nitamba
Indravasti	

Vishalyaghna Marmas

These are called Vishalyaghna because the points need regular and lifelong treatment to live (Yapya).

Utkshep	Sthapni

Vaikalyakar Marm:

These are called Vaikalyakar because there is loss and impairment of any part of body or organ such as in Poliomyelitis, muscular atrophy, hemiplegia:

Lohitaksha
Janu
Urvi
Kurch
Vitap
Kurpar
Ans
Ansphalak
Apang
Neel
Manya
Fan
Kukundar
Kakshadhar
Vidhur
Krikatika
Avarta

Rujakar Marm

Pain, Motor impairment and muscular atrophy are prominent features of Rujakar Marm.

Gulph
Kurchshir
Manibandh

Chapter 7

LOCATION AND INDICATION OF MARMAS

Mans Marmas

Talhridaya Marmas (Figures 21, 22)
Acharya Sushrut mentions:

मध्यमाङ्गुलीमनुपूर्वेण मध्ये पादतलस्य तलहृदयं नाम, तत्र रुजाभिर्मरणं

(सु०शा०, 6/24)

Madhyamangulimanupurven madhye padtalasya talhridayamnam, tatra rujabhirmaranam

(Sushrut Sharir, 6/24)

The Talhridaya Marm lies on the centre of the line drawn between the middle finger and centre of palm or sole. According to the location these are called Sakthi Marm (Marmas of extremities).

The total number of Talhridaya Marm are four. Two in upper extremity and two in lower extremity.

1. Name of the Marm	Talhridaya
2. Type of Marm	Mans Marm
3. Prognosis	Kalantar Pranhar (Fatal after some time)
4. Quality-Somya/Agneya	Somya+Agneya
5. Size	Half Angul (1.0-1.5 cms)
6. Location	In the centre of the line drawn between middle finger and centre of Palm or Sole. Tallhridaya 8-P8 + Hridaya 8-H8,Vrikka1-K1 (Figures 21, 22)
7. Indications	Cardiac Pain (Pain is the prominent Symptom)

The Talhridaya Marmas are Mans Marma and according to Sushrut Sharir 26/40—when the Mans Marmas are afflicted, the patient has sensory loss of the particular area and the colour becomes dusty pale (Paṇdu Varn). All Mans Marmas carry two distinct fibres - one to stop pain and the other to stop bleeding.

According to *Sushrut Sharir*, 6/32:

क्षिप्रेषु तत्र सतलेषु.......

(सु०शा०, 6/32)

Kshipreshu tatra sataleshu.......

Heavy loss of blood from the particular organ causes increase in Vata neurohumour resulting in severe pain. There are two marms under it: Talhridaya of hand and Talhridaya of foot which are having P8 and K1 points respectively. Stimulation of these points stops pain and bleeding. One of the main causes of pain related to this Marm is acute Myocardial Infarction and Angina (Cardiac Pain). So this can be checked by stimulation of these two points specially P8 and their regular prophylatic use definitely cures angina pain and helps in reducing the frequency and severity of attack.

VRIKKA DHAMANI AND TAL HRIDAYA MARMAS OF SAKTHI (Lower Extremity) (Kaphaj - Stri Sangyak) K : KIDNEY CHANNEL (Yin)

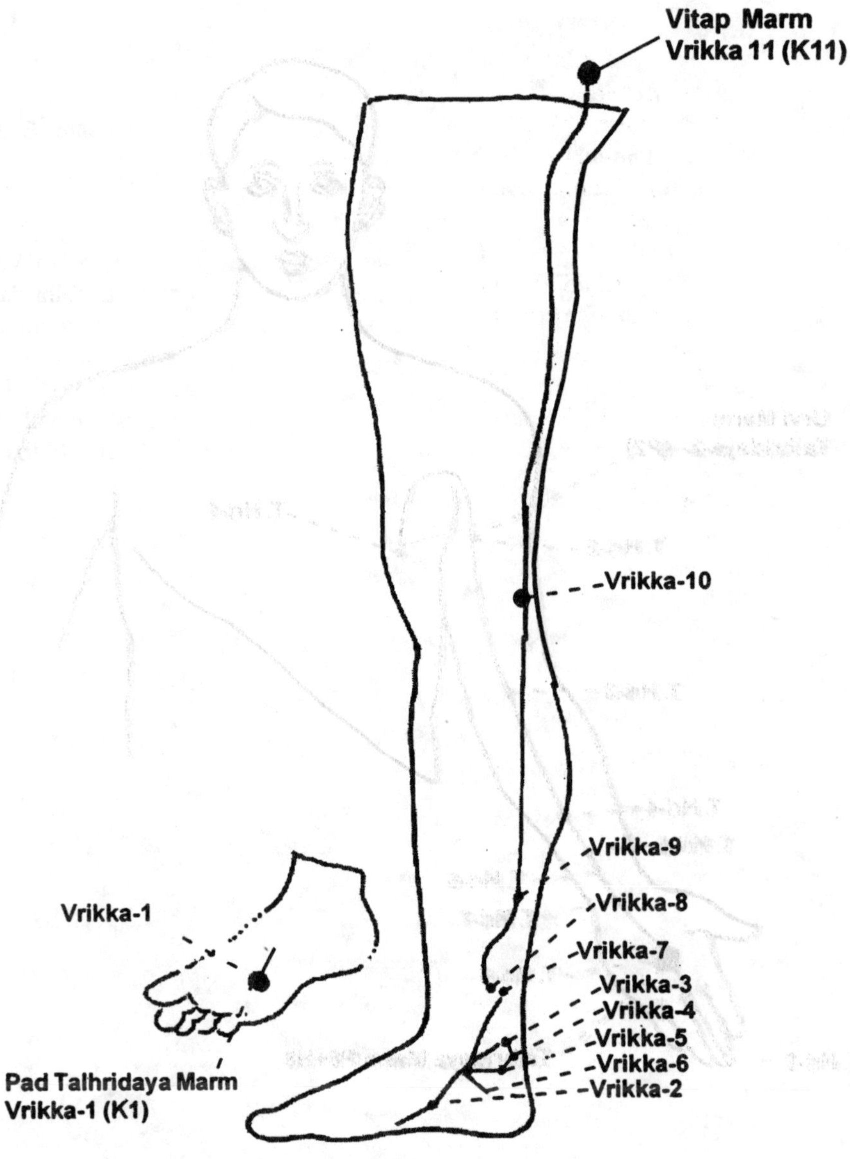

Figure 21

P: PERICARDIUM CHANNEL (Yin)
TRIYAGA TAL HRIDAYA DHAMANI, MARM AND SIRA OF UPPER EXTREMITIES

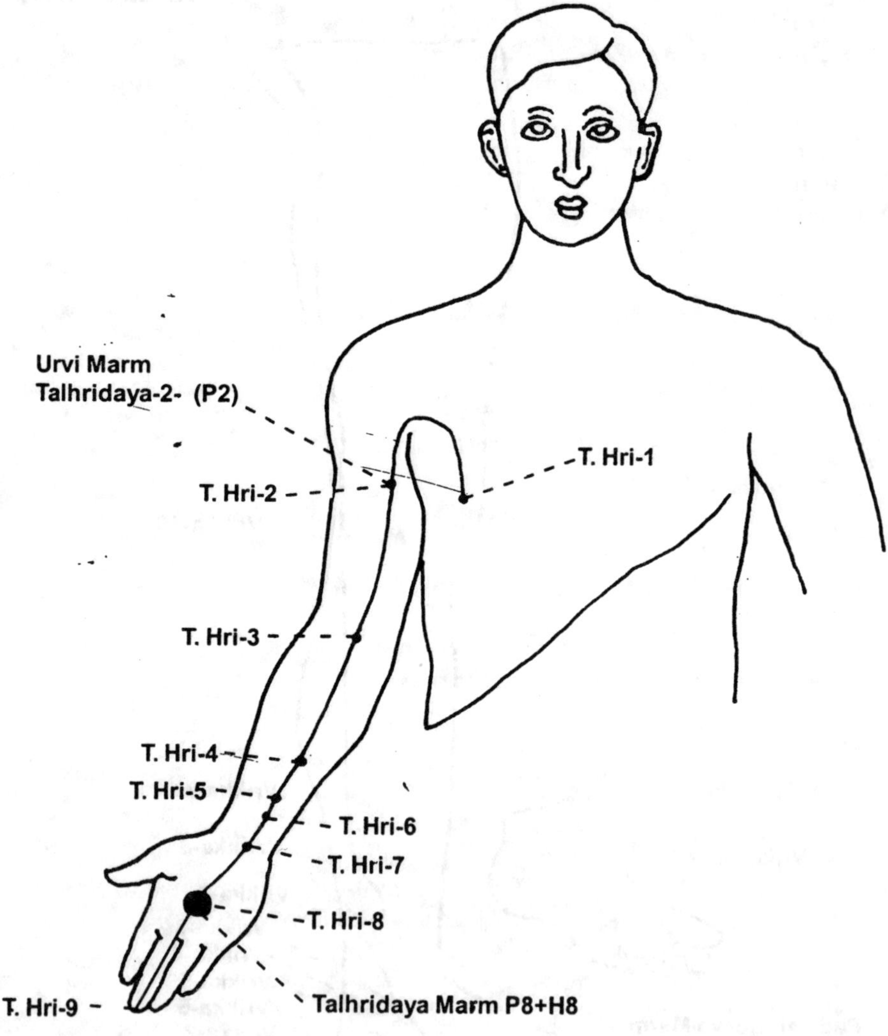

Figure 22

Indra Vasti Marmas: (See Figures 23, 24)
Acharya Sushrut mentions:

पार्ष्णि प्रति जङ्घामध्ये इन्द्रवस्तिः ।
तत्र शोणितक्षयेण मरणं ।।

(सु०शा०, 6/24)

Parshni prati Janghamadhye Indravbastih,
Tatra Shonit Kshayen Marnam.

(Su. Sharir, 6/24)

This Marm lies in the centre of calf muscle.
According to location these are called Sakthi Marm. The total number of Indravasti Marmas are four. Two in upper extremity and two in lower extremity.

1. Name of the Marm	Indrabasti
2. Type of Marm	Mans Marm
3. Prognosis	Kalantar Pranhar (fatal after sometime) Death due to blood loss after sometime.
4. Quality (Agneya/ Somya)	Somya+Agneya
5. Size	Half Angul (1.0-1.5 cms)
6. Location	Lower Extremity: In the centre of the calf muscle in leg Mutrashaya 58-UB58+ Pittashaya 35 - GB 35. Upper Extremity: In the centre and anterior of the fore arm Talhridaya 4- P4, Phuffus 6-Lu6 (Figures 23, 24)
7. Indications	*Shonitkshayen marnam (Su.Sh., 6/24)* Death due to loss of blood from any part of the body i.e.—Haemoptysis, Hemetemesis, Haemorrhoids, Epistaxis etc.

INDRA VASTI MARM & MUTRASHAY DHAMANI UB CHANNEL (Yang)

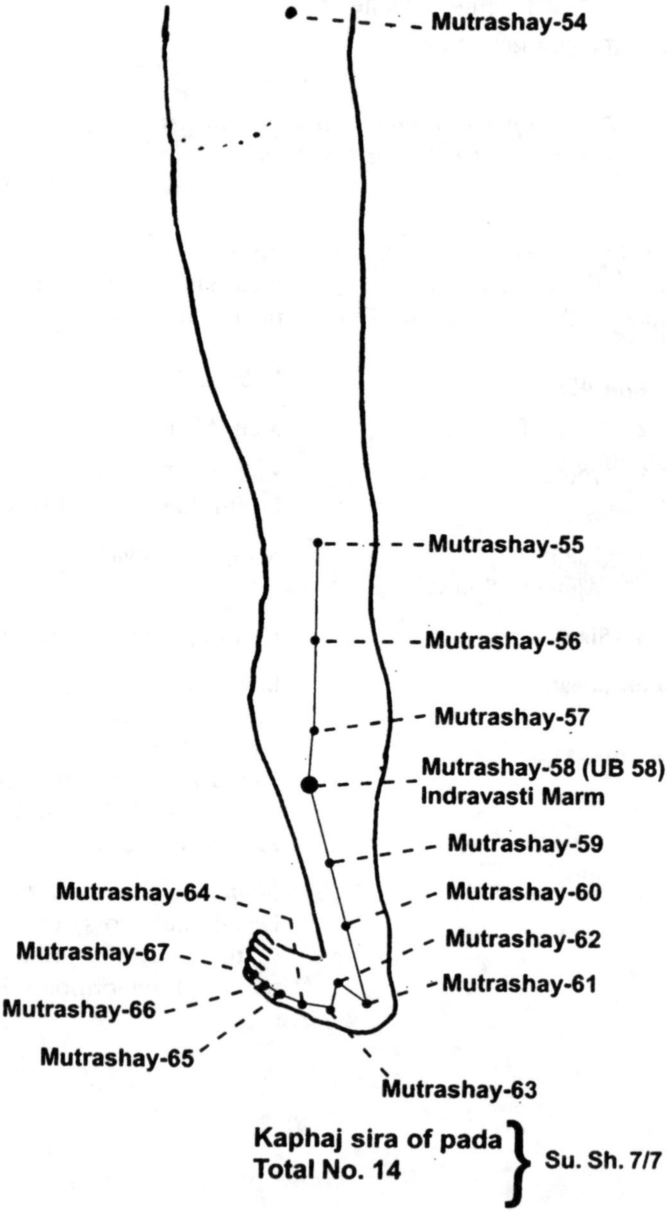

Figure 23

INDRAVASTI MARM AND URDHVAGA PHUFFUS DHAMANI & VATAJ SIRA OF HAND
Lu: Lung Channel (Yin)

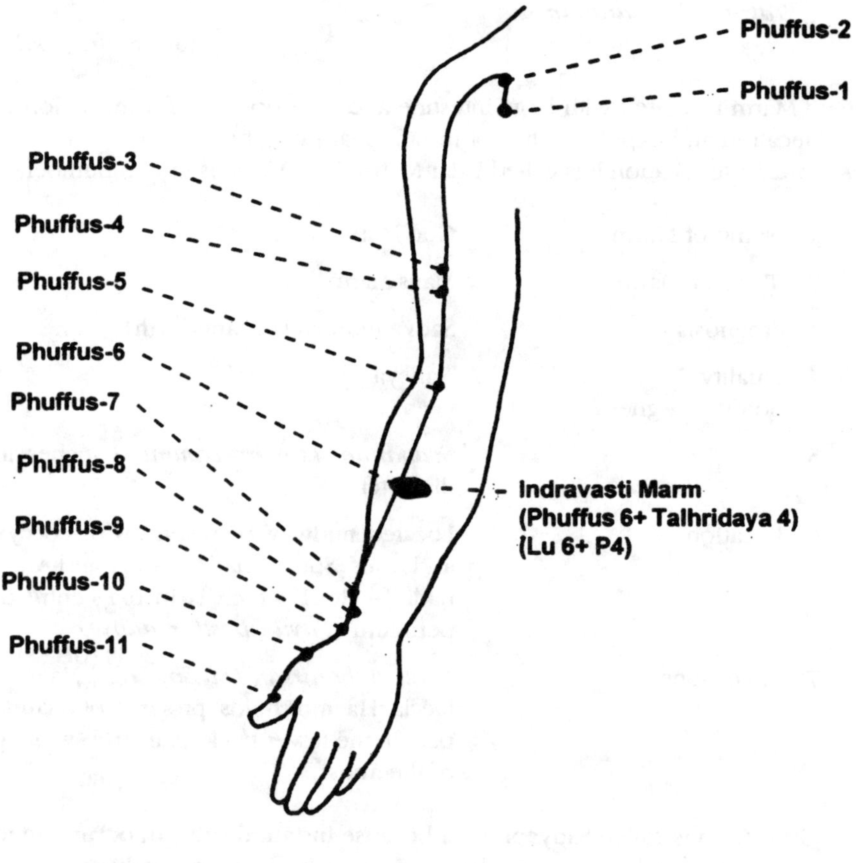

Figure 24

Gud Marm: (Figure 25)

Acharya Sushrut says:

तत्र वातवर्चोनिरसन स्थूलान्त्रप्रतिबद्धं गुद नाम मर्म, तत्र सद्योमरणम्।

(सु०शा०, 6/25)

Tatra Vat-varchonirasan sthulantrapratibaddham Gud nam Marm Tatra sadyomaranam.

(Su. Sharir, 6/25)

Gud Marm is related with large intestine and is responsible for the action of defaecation and expulsion. It is of instant death variety.

According to location it is called Udar Marm. This Marm is one in number.

1. Name of Marm.	Gud Marm
2. Type of Marm	Mans Marm
3. Prognosis	Sadya pranhar (instant death)
4. Quality Somya / Agneya	Agneya
5. Size	*Svapanital kunchit sammit* 2 inches in diameter
6. Location	Located midway between tip of coccyx and Anus. Shukra nadi 1—Du1 and Artav nadi 1—Ren1 which is in the centre of perinium *(Payu upasth madhye)*
7. Indications	*(Vatvarchonirsan (Su.Sh. 6/25)* Haema-faecia, Haemorrhoids, prolapse of rectum, pain in the lower back, pain and swelling of the anus:

Gud Marm is called Sadyapranhar because instant death can occur due to vaso-vagal shock during manipulation of organ in certain procedures. As it is Agneya, the fire element cools rapidly and death occurs. The above mentioned pain is due to manipulation during operation of fissure, piles and fistula. The pain subsides immediately on sitz bath by the stimulation of the Guda Marm points Du1, Ren1 (2 inches in diameter *(Svapanital kunchit)*. This Marm is of great importance for Anorectal Surgeons. For prolapse of rectum, haemorrhoids and fissure, the Guda Marm points Ren1, and Du1, should be stimulated either by needle or by heat.

ARTAV NADI AND HRIDAYA, NABHI, VASTI & GUD MARM
(Ren channel - Extra channel)

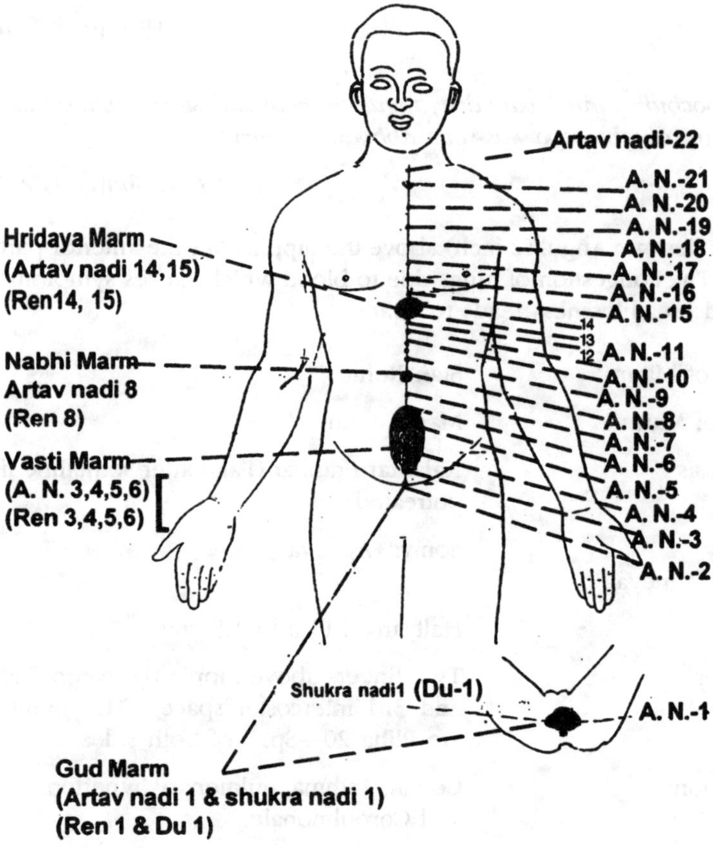

6 Pittaj and raktaj sira of udar (Abdomen) S. Sh. 7/7

Figure 25

Stan Rohit (Figure 26)

According to location it is called Vaksh Marm (Marm of Chest).

स्तनचूचुकयोरुर्ध्वंद्वयङ्गुलमुभयतः स्तनरौहितौ, तत्र
लोहितपूर्णकोष्ठतया कासश्वासाभ्यां च म्रियते।

(सु०शा०, 6/25)

Stanchoochukayorurdhvam dvayangulamubhayatah stanrouhitou tatra Lohitpoornakoshthtaya kas-shvasabhyam ch mriyate

(Su. Sharir, 6/25)

This Marm lies two Angul (2 inch) above the nipple over the anterior part of the chest. The congestion of lungs due to blood which causes symptoms of cough and breathlessness leads to death.

1. Name of Marm	Stan Rohit
2. Type of Marm	Mans Marm
3. Prognosis	Kalantar Pranhar (Fatal after sometime if untreated)
4. Quality Somya/Agneya	Somya+Agneya
5. Size	Half angul (1.0 to 1.5 cms)
6. Location	Two fingers above nipple (between 2nd and 3rd intercostal space). The points are Pliha 20—Sp20 of both sides.
7. Indication	Cough, Asthma, pulmonary hypertension and Corpulmonale.

These points should be stimulated to cure the above mentioned diseases either by Agnikarm (Moxibustion) or acupuncture (Siravedhan). For prophylatic uses the stimulation may be continued for a longer duration. The prominent symptom of involvement of this Marm is heavy breathing caused by fulness of chest due to accumulation of blood (Su. Sh. 6/25). In worst cases the Mastitis may be due to malignancy.

SIRA, DHAMANI AND MARM OF KOSHTH (TORSO)

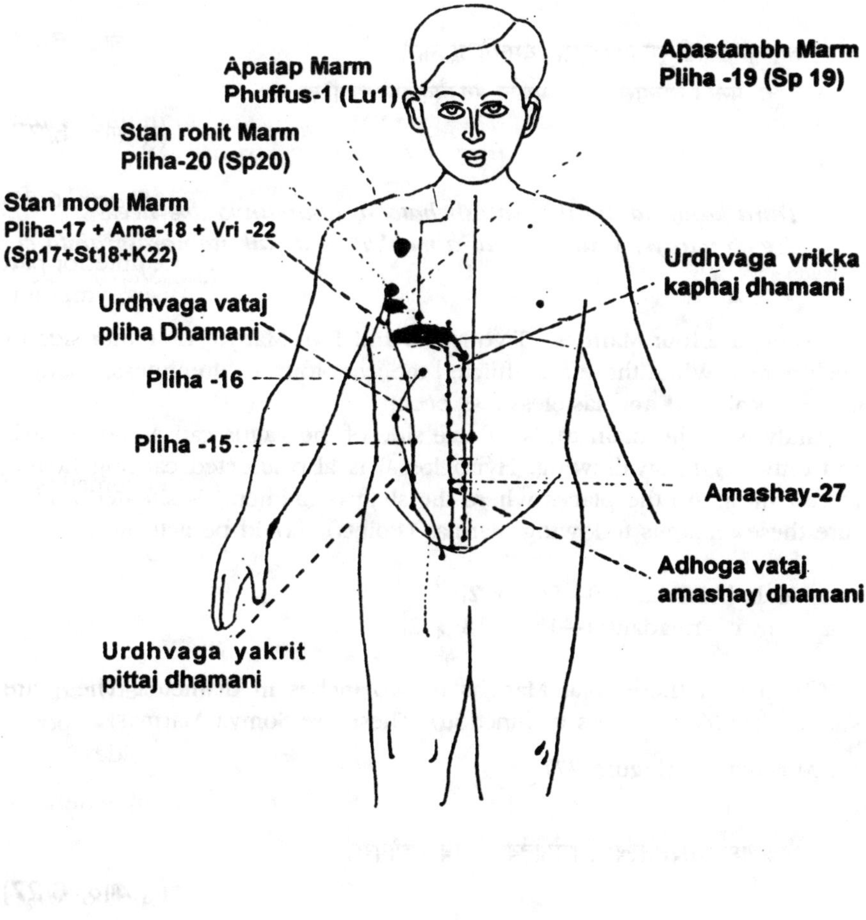

Figure 26

Sira Marmas (Figure 27)

(1) Neel Dhamani (Manya + Neel Dhamani) : These are the marm of *Urdhvajatru* (Above the clavicle)

According to Su.Sh. 6/27

तत्र कण्ठनाड़ीमुभयतश्चतस्रो धमन्यो द्वे नीले
द्वे च मन्ये। व्यत्यासेन तत्र मूकता स्वरवैकृतमरसग्राहिता च।

(सु०शा०, 6/27)

Tatra kanthnadimubhayatashchatasro dhamanyo dve neele
dve ch manye, Vyatyasen tatra mookata svarvaikritamarasgrahita ch.
(Su. Sharir., 6/27)

There are four Marmas - Two Neela and Two Manyas on either side of the Trachea. When these are afflicted the symptoms of dumbness, changes in the vocal cord and tastelessness occur.

Paralysis of the main trunk of one side of the vagus causes hoarseness and difficulty in swallowing. Hypoglossal is also affected causing hoarse voice - these are the places where the shalyas (ailment) is situated and to cure these ailments following Marmas (Points) should be activated:

2 Neela [Amashaya 9—St 9 x 2]
2 Manya [Vrihadantra—18 LI 18 x 2]

The size of these total Marmas is two inches in diameter. These are Vaikalyakar Marms (Loss of function). These are Somya Marmas.

(2) Matrika - 8 (Figure 27)

ग्रीवायामुभयतश्चतस्त्रः सिरामातृकाः, तत्र सद्योमरणं

(सु०शा०, 6/27)

Greevayamubhyatashchatasrahsiramatrikah tatra sadhyomaranam
(Su. Sharir, 6/27)

This is Urdhvajatru Marm (point above clavicle). According to *Su.Sh.* 6/27, on either side of neck there are four Sira Matrikas. When these are damaged instant death occurs.

These points are debatable and following are the possibilities:

(a) The instant death may be due to Carotid Sinus Syncope.

(b) These 8 Matrikas are not related to points of regular channels but probably these may be point of extra channels.

(c) Possible points may be from Ren and Du channels because the word, Ubhay in the shlok may indicate anterior and posterior part of the neck.

(d) According to dictionary, Matrika, in Sanskrit means necklace and following points make the necklace:

Artavnadi 23	— Ren 23	
Shukra nadi 15	— Du 15	
Pittashaya 21	— GB 21	of both sides — Total 8 Points.
Shleshmashay 16	— Sj 16	of both sides — Total 8 Points.
Vrihadantra 17	— LI 17	of both sides — Total 8 Points.

These are Sadyapranhar Marms.

MARM, PITTAVAHINI DHAMANI AND SIRA OF URDHVAJATRU (ABOVE CLAVICLE)

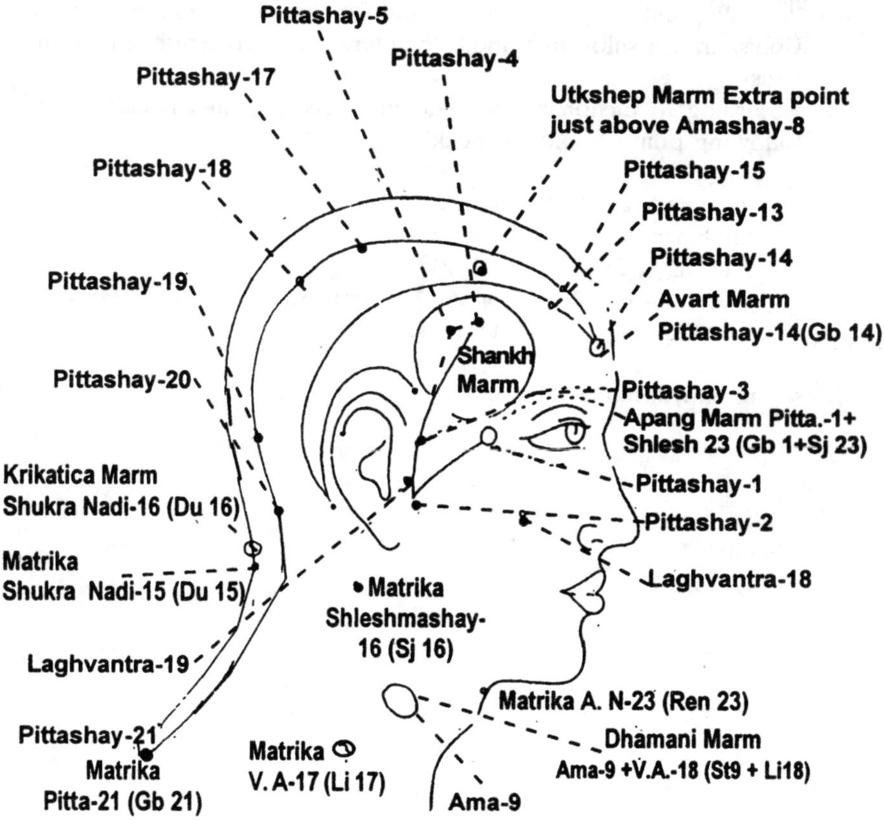

Figure 27

Shringatak Marm (Figure 28)

These are four in number - two on either side of head.

घ्राणश्रोत्राक्षिजिह्वसंतर्पणीनां सिराणां मध्ये
सिरा सन्निपातः श्रृङ्गाटकानि

(सु० शा०, 6/27)

Ghran shrotakshi jihva santarpaninam siranam
Madhye sira sannipatah shringatakani

(Sushrut Sharir, 6/27)

In between the meeting point of Siras which nourish nose, eyes, ear and tongue are called Shringatak Marms. (Santarpan : Nourish (poshan) (*Su.Sh.*, 9/5)

1. Name of Marm	Shringatak Marm
2. Type of Marm	Sira Marm
3. Prognosis	Sadya pranhar
4. Quality Somya/Agneya	Agneya
5. Size	Svapanital kunchit (2 inches in diameter)
6. Location	Head
7. Indication	Death due to Intracranial Haemorrhage

First Shringatak has following points (x2 both sides)

Pittashay 4	— GB 4	—	Nourishes eyes
Amashay 8	— ST 8	—	Nourishes smell and taste
Mutrashay4	— UB 4	—	Nourishes ears

The Shringatak Marm is present in between the meeting points of the above Siras. At the junction of these three points a figure of horn is formed.

Second Shringatak has the following points x2

Pittashay15	— GB 15	— Nourishes eyes
Mutrashay5	— UB 5	— Nourishes ears
Shukra nadi 22, 23	— Du 22, 23	— Nourishes smell and taste

This marm is situated in between the junction of the above three points. Another Shring is formed at the junction of these three points. The disease of this marm is situated in the hypothalamus and pituitary. Haemorrhage occurs either by accident or postpartum or any growth which causes shock

SHRINGATAK MARM

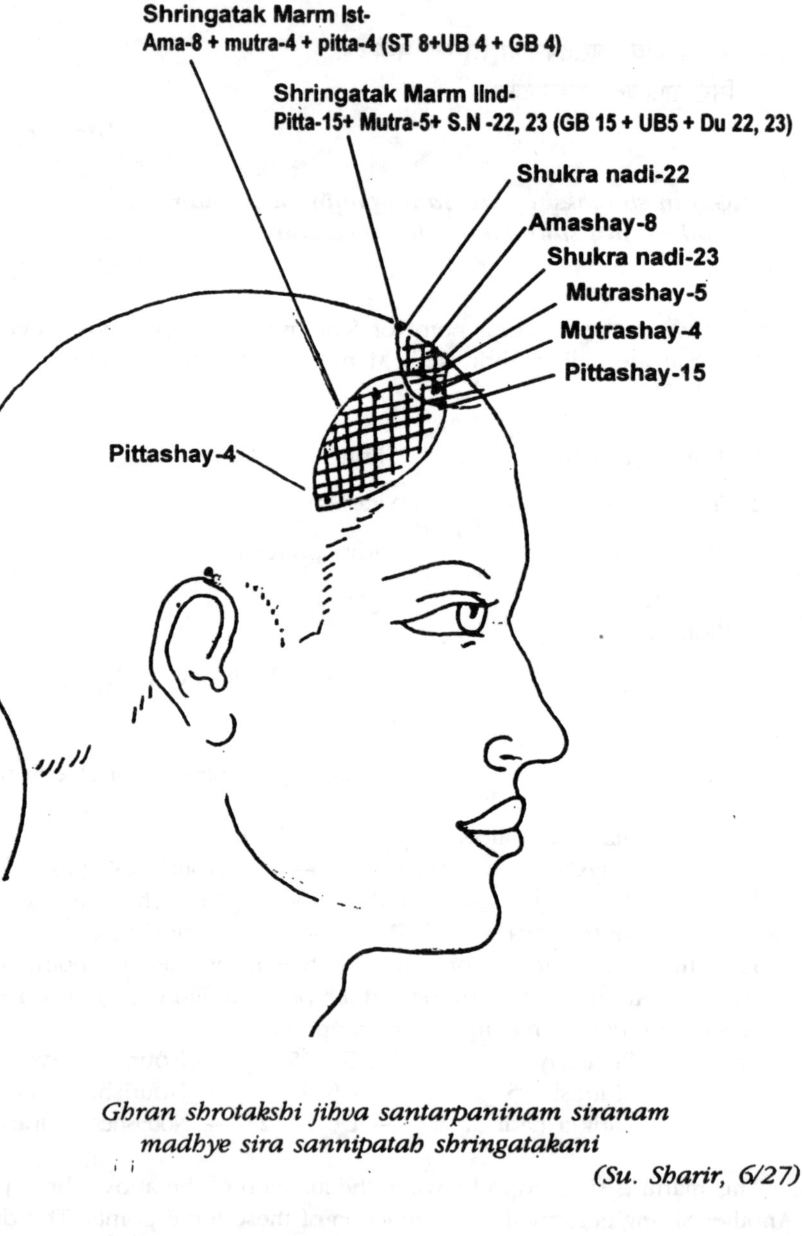

Ghran shrotakshi jihva santarpaninam siranam
madhye sira sannipatah shringatakani

(Su. Sharir, 6/27)

Figure 28

and hypothermia. The other causes of Intracranial haemorrhages which occur in the following places as thalamic haemorrhage, pontine haemorrhage and cerebellar haemorrhage. It occurs in the following conditions:

1. Hypertensive cerebral Haemorrhage
2. Ruptured Sacular Aneurysm
3. Haemorrhage associated with bleeding disorders
4. Intracranial Haemorrhage due to head injuries

On the onset of symptoms the treatment should be started by immediate stimulation of these four marmas. The earlier the procedure is initiated the better are the results.

Explanation:

Pittashay 4, 15 — GB 4 and GB 15 : These are agni points to stop blood by constricting the veins due to Dah Kriya.

दाहः संकोचयेत् सिरा,

(सु०सू०, 14/40)

Dahah sankochyet sira,

(Su. Sutra, 14/40)

Mutrashay 4, 5 — UB4, and UB5: These are jal points, coagulates blood due to its cold action (Him Kriya)

रक्तं स्कंदयते हिमम्

(सु०सू०, 14/40)

Raktam skandayte himam

(Su.Sutra, 14/40)

Amashay 8, Shukranadi 22, 23 — ST8, DU22—23 :These are vayu points leading to *Astringent* (Kashay) action.

कषायः संधते

(सु०सू०, 14/40)

Kashayah sandhate

(Su. Sutra, 14/40)

Apang Marm (Figure 29)

These are two in number. These are marm of Urdhvajatru (Above Clavicle)

भ्रूपुच्छांतयोरधोऽक्ष्णोर्बाह्यतोऽपांङ्गौ तत्रान्ध्यं दृष्ट्युपघातो वा

(सु० शा०, 6/27)

Bhrupuchantayoradhoakshanorbahyatoapangou tatrandhyam dristyupghato va

(Śu. Sharir, 6/27)

1.	Name of Marm	Apang
2.	Type of Marm	Sira marm
3.	Prognosis	Vaikalyakar (may cause blindness)
4.	Quality Somya/Agneya	Somya + Agneya
5.	Size	Half Angul (1.0-1.5 cms)
6.	Location	Just below the end of eyebrows. The points are Pittashay 1 and Shleshmashay 23 (GB 1 and Sj 23)
7.	Indication	*Bhrupuchantayoradhoakshano....... Tatrandhyam drishty upghato va* Blurring of vision, blindness.

Explanation :

Stimulation of point Pittashay 1 (GB 1), reduces the redness of eye by absorbing blood clot and consequently improves the vision. Stimulation of Shleshmashay 23 (Sj 23) will have a similar action. Sushrut has contra-indicated acupuncture to Apang Sira. (*Sushrut Sharir,* 7/22)

According to Sushrut, stimulation by kshar and agni is best for Apang Marm. Kshar is prepared mainly from lime and mokha tree.

MARM, PITTAVAHINI DHAMANI AND SIRA OF URDHVAJATRU (ABOVE CLAVICLE)

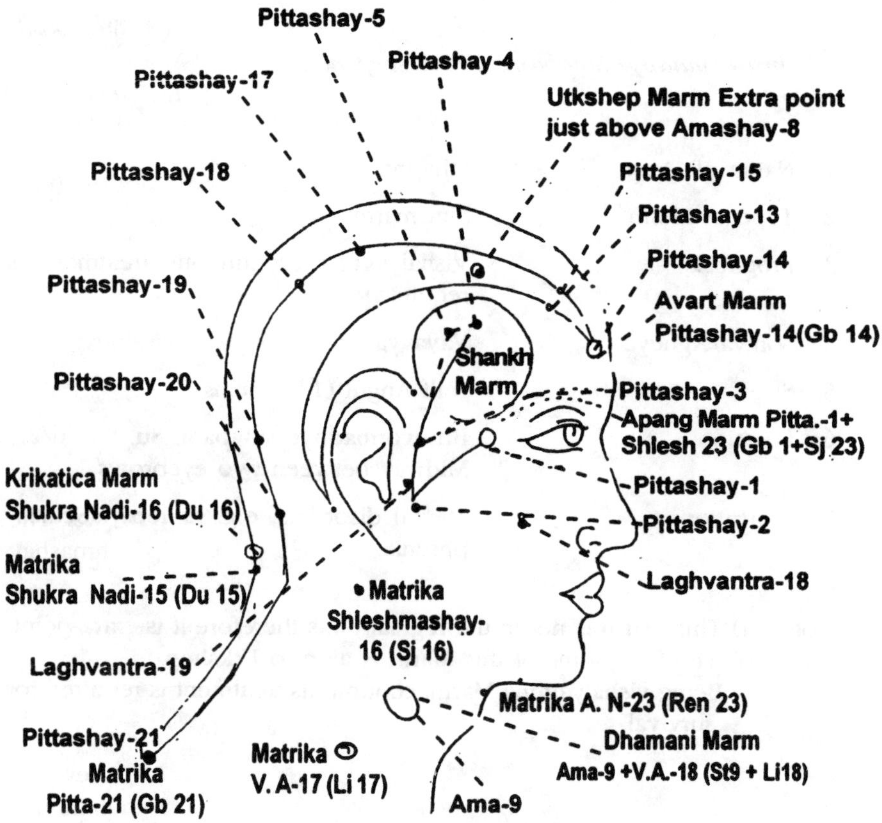

Figure 29

Sthapani Marm (Figure 30)

This Marm is single in number and this is the Marm of Urdhvajatru (above the clavicle)

भ्रुवोर्मध्ये स्थपनी, तत्रोत्क्षेपवत्।

(सु०शा०, 6/27)

Bhruvormadhye Sthapani, Tatrotkshepvat.

(Su. Sharir, 6/27)

1.	Name of Marm	Sthapni
2.	Type of Marm	Sira marm
3.	Prognosis	Vishalyaghna (continuous treatment is required)
4.	Somya/Agneya	Vayavya
5.	Size	Half Angul (1.0-1.5cms)
6.	Location	Bhruvormadhyc sthapani, Su. Sh., 6/27 Midway between two eyebrows
7.	Indications	Mental disorders, e.g. Epilepsy, Schizophrenia.

Note: (a) This Marm is not in the regular Siras therefore it is extra point.
(b) The Symptoms of this Marm is akin to Utkshep.
(c) Being vishalyaghna Marm, continuous treatment is required for survival.

VATAJ, PITTAJ DHAMANI AND SIRAS OF GREEVA (NECK) FAN AND STHAPNI MARM

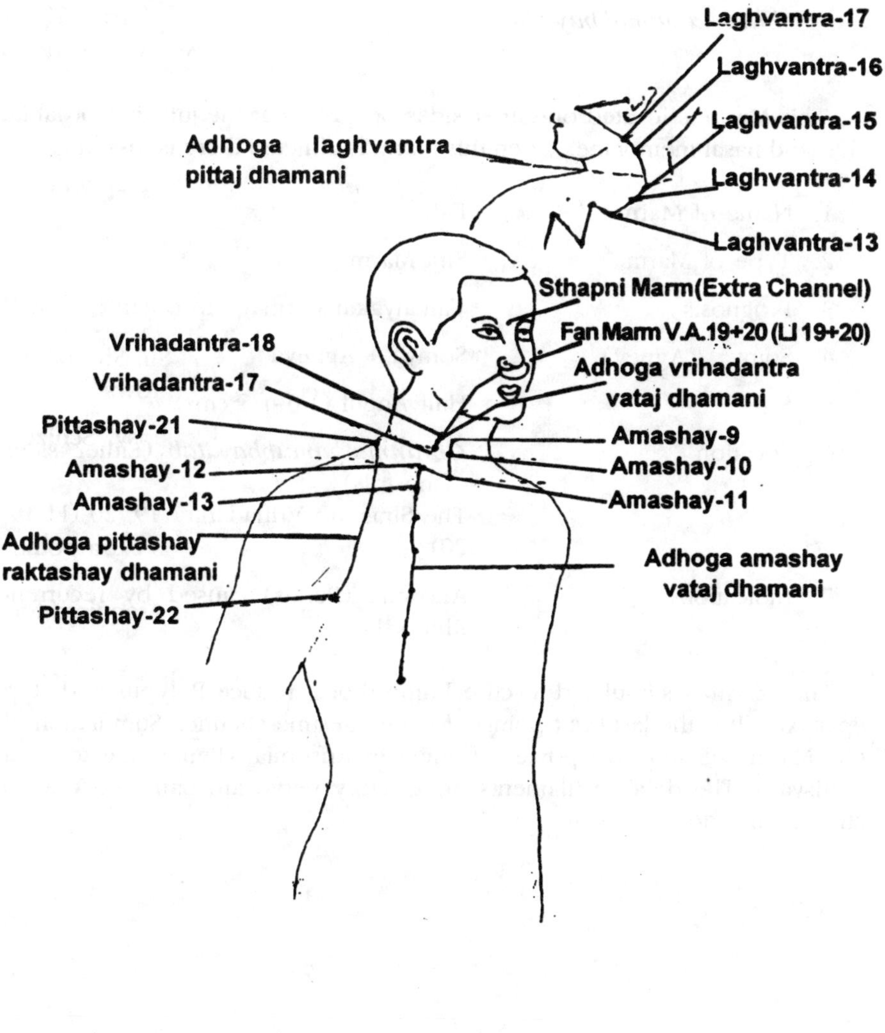

Figure 30

Fan Marm (Figure 31)

This is also Urdhvajatru Marm (above clavicle)

घ्राणमार्गमुभयतः

(सु०शा०, 6/27)

Ghranmargamubhayatah

(Su. Sharir, 6/27)

This Marm is located on either sides of nostrils at the junction of labial skin and nasal membrane. When this Marm is afflicted there is loss of smell.

1. Name of Marm	Fan
2. Type of Marm	Sira Marm
3. Prognosis	Vaikalyakar (damage to organ of smell)
4. Somya / Agneya	Somya + Agneya
5. Size	Half Angul (1.0–1.5 cms)
6. Location	*Ghranmargamubhayatah* (Either sides of nostrils) The Siras are Vrihadantra 19, 20 (LI 19, 20)
7. Indications	Anosmia (Penus) caused by recurrent Rhinorrhoea

This Marm is stimulated to cure Rhinorrhoea, reduce Polypus and stop epistaxis. It is the last (exit point) of large intestine channel. Stimulation of this Marm will improve power of smell in Ansomia. (Penus due to Jirna Pratisyay). The delicate filaments of olfactory nerve are damaged due to chronic infections.

VATAJ, PITTAJ DHAMANI AND SIRAS OF GREEVA (NECK) FAN AND STHAPNI MARM

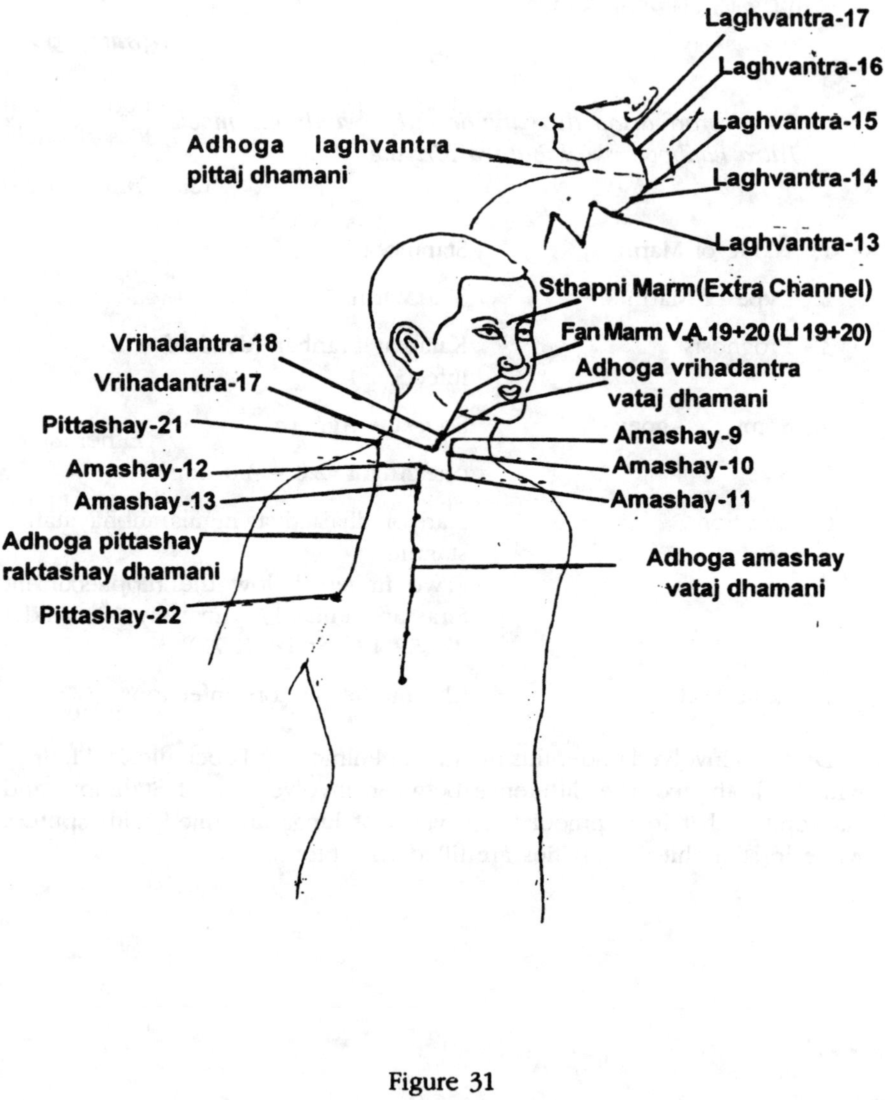

Figure 31

Stan mool (Figure 32)

This is Vaksha Marm (Marm of Chest). According to Sushrut, the marm lies at the base of lungs two fingers below the nipples. In chronic respiratory infections death may occur due to filling of cough and sputum in these Marms.

स्तनयोरधस्ताद् द्वयङ्गुलमुभयतः स्तनमूले
तत्र कफपूर्णकोष्ठतया म्रियते।

(सु०शा०, 6/25)

Stanayoradhastad dvayangulamubhayatah Stanmoole
Tatra kaphpoornkoshthataya Mriyate

(Su. Sharir, 6/25)

1. Name of Marm	Stanmool
2. Type of Marm	Sira Marm
3. Prognosis	Kalantar Pranhar (death due to chronic infections)
4. Somya / Agneya	Somya + Agneya
5. Size	one Angul (2.0 – 3.0 Cms)
6. Location	Stanyoradhastadvayangulamubhayatah stanmule (Two fingers below the nipples). The Siras are: Pliha 17, Amashay 18, Vrikka 22 (SP 17, St 18, K 22)
7. Indications	Chronic Respiratory infections

Diseases involved under this marm are: Pulmonary Tuberculosis, Pleurisy with Hydrothorax. The difference between involvement of Stanmool and Stanrohit is that in stanmool the cavities of lungs are filled with sputum while in stanrohit the cavities are filled with blood.

SIRA, DHAMANI AND MARM OF TORSO AND ABDOMEN (KOSHTHAGAT)

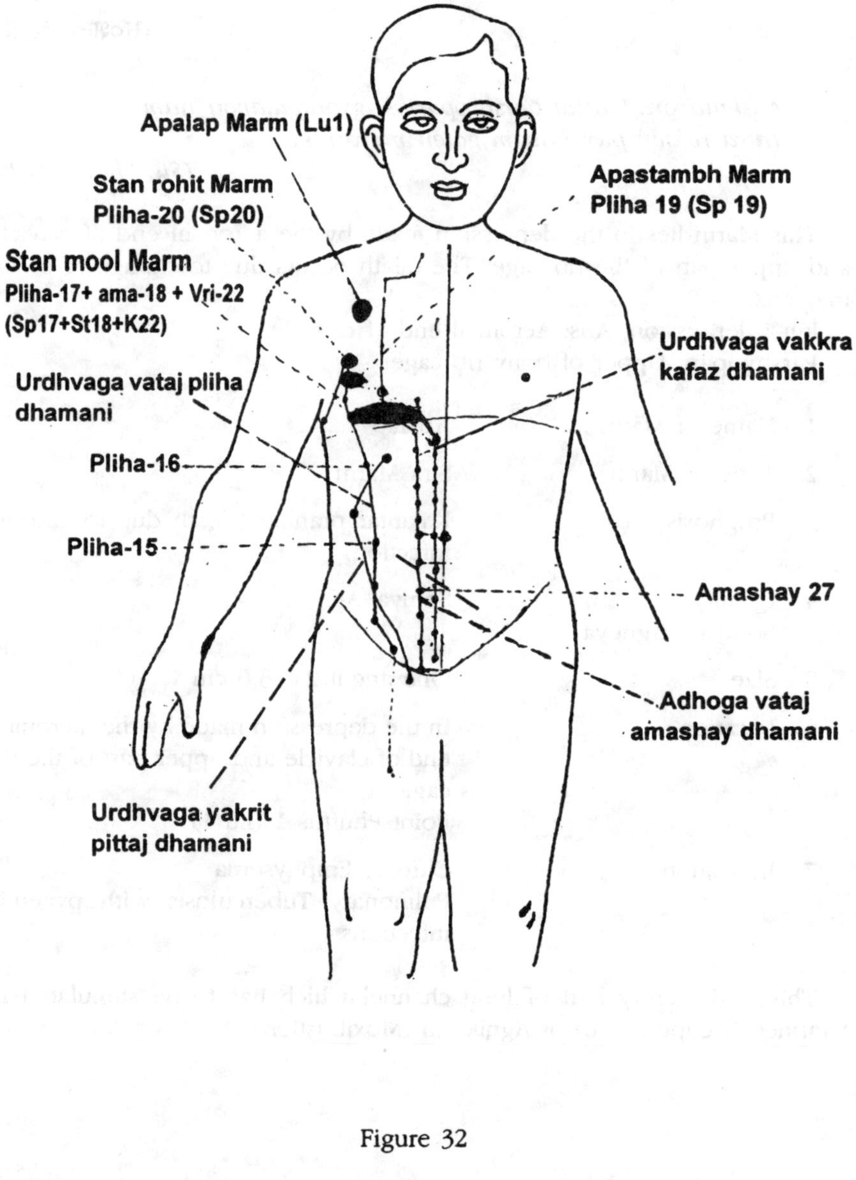

Figure 32

Apalap Marm (Figure 33)

This is also Vaksha marm(The marm of chest). According to Shusrut,

अंसकूटयोरधस्तात् पार्श्वोपरिभागयोरपलापौ नाम
तत्र रक्तेन पूयभावं गतेन मरणं

(सु०शा०, 6/25)

Anskutayoradhastat parshvoparibhagyorapalapou nam
Tatra rakten puybhavam gaten maranam

(Su. Sharir, 6/25)

This Marm lies in the depression made by the acromial end of clavicle and upper part of the rib cage. The death occurs due to change of blood into pus.

kut : depression, Ans: Acromial end of clavicle.
Parshvopari: Upper of bony rib cage.

1. Name of Marm	Apalap
2. Type of Marm	Sira Marm
3. Prognosis	Kalantar pranhar (death due to chronic infection)
4. Quality Somya / Agneya	Somya+Agneya
5. Size	One angul 2.0–3.0 cm
6. Location	In the depression made by the acromial end of clavicle and upper part of the rib cage. Point Phuffus 1 (Lu 1)
7. Indications	Chronic Emphysema Pulmonary Tuberculosis with pyaemic infections

This is the entry part of lung channel which has to be stimulated in Sirabhed (Acupuncture) or Agnikarm (Moxibustion).

SIRA, DHAMANI AND MARM OF TORSO AND ABDOMEN (KOSHTHAGAT)

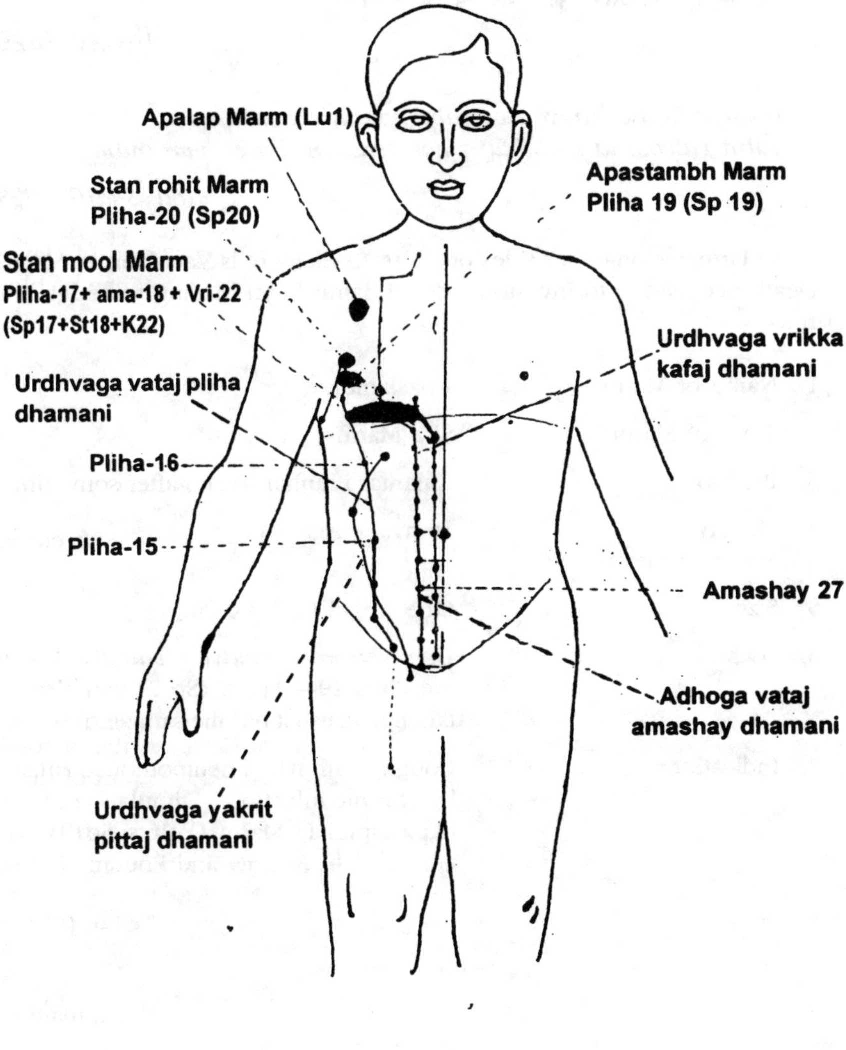

Figure 33

Apastambh Marm (Figure 34)

This is also Vaksha Marm (The marm of chest). According to *S.Sh.*, 6/25.

उभयत्रोरसो नाड्यौ वातवहे अपस्तम्भौ नाम,
तत्र वातपूर्ण कोष्ठतया कासश्वासाभ्यां च मरणं।।

(सु०शा०, 6/25)

Ubhayatroraso nadyou vatvahe apastambhou nam
Tatra vatpoorna koshthtaya kasshvasabhyam ch maranam

(Su. Sharir, 6/25)

This Marm lies on either sides of chest. Its element is Vata (Saman Vayu). Death occurs due to invasion of cold damp Vayu leading to cough and Asthma.

1. Name of Marm	Apastambh
2. Type of Marm	Sira Marm
3. Prognosis	Kalantar Pranhar (death after some time)
4. Quality Somya/Agneya	Somya + Agneya
5. Size	One Angul (2.0–3.0 cm)
6. Location	*Ubhayatroraso nadyou vatvahe* Points are Pliha 19— Sp 19 (Sp 21 can also be taken because it has the same indication).
7. Indications	Cough, Asthmā Pneumothorax caused by chronic infections. Stimulation of this (Apastambha) Marm (Points Sp19) will cure cough, Asthma and Pneumothorax.

SIRA, DHAMANI AND MARM OF TORSO AND ABDOMEN (KOSHTHAGAT)

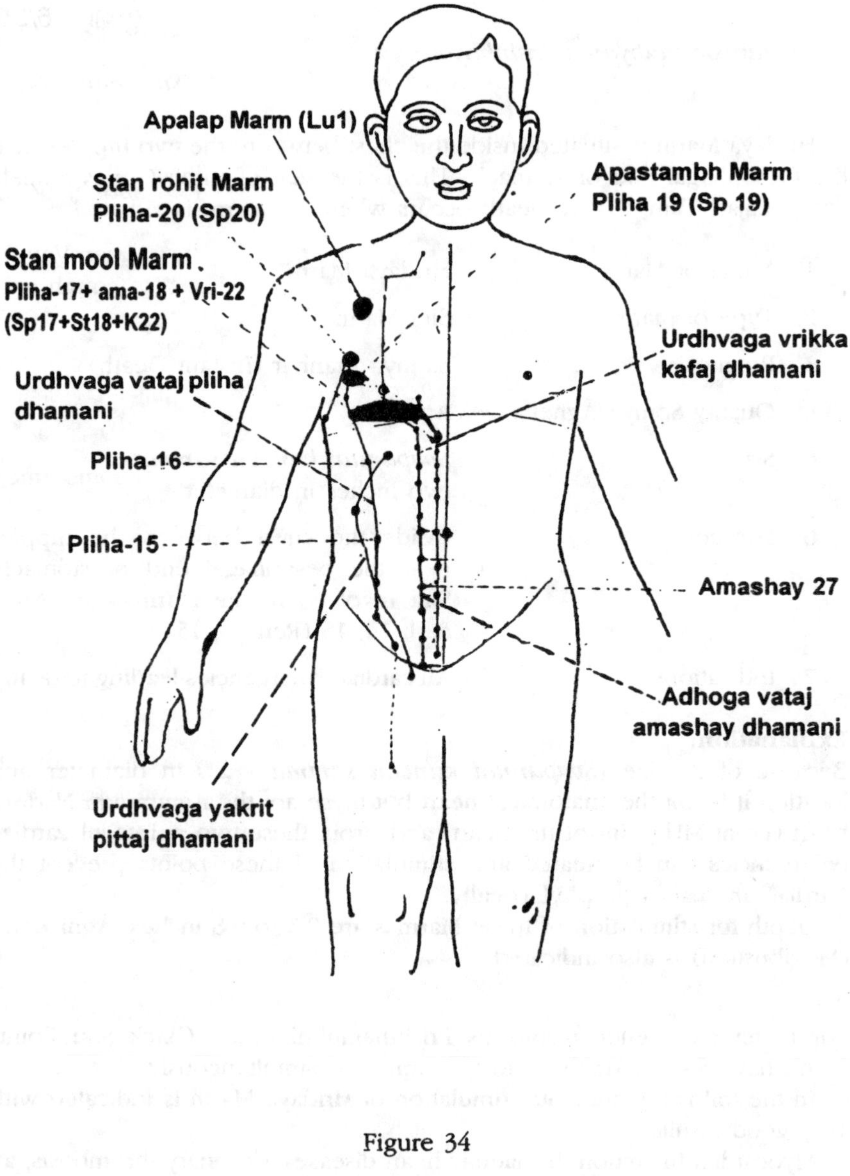

Figure 34

Hridaya Marm (Figure 35)

This is also included in Sira Marm and is a Single Marm. According to *Su. Sh.*, 6/25:

स्तनयोर्मध्यमधिष्ठायोरस्य...........

(सु०शा०, 6/25)

Stanyormadhyamadhishthayorasya ....

(Su. Sharir, 6/25)

Hridaya Marm is situated inside the chest between the two nipples near the Oesophagal end of stomach. This is the seat of three Gunas namely Satva, Rajas, Tam. Instant death occurs when the marm is afflicted.

1. Name of Marm	Hridaya Marm
2. Type of Marm	Sira Marm
3. Prognosis	Sadhya Pranhar (Instant Death)
4. Quality Somya/Agneya	Agneya
5. Size	*Svapanital kunchit sammit* two inches in diameter
6. Location	Inside the chest between the nipples near the oesophagal end of stomach. Sira involved in the Marmas are Artav nadi 14, 15 (Ren 14, 15).
7. Indications	All cardiac emergencies leading to death.

Explanation:

Because of its size *(Svapanital kunchit sammit - 2")* in diameter and location it is not the anatomical heart but these are the Agramukhi Nadi of heart (Front MU point of the heart) and from these two points all cardiac emergencies can be treated and stimulation of these points prevent the Cardiac anomalies prophylactically.

Depth for stimulation of these Marmas are 0.3 to 0.8 inches. Agni Karm (Moxibustion) is also indicated.

Note:

For better therapeutic results its Prishthamukhi Bindu (Back Shu Point) Mutrashay 15— (UB15) should be stimulated simultaneously.

In the following ailments stimulation of Hridaya Marm is indicated with very good results:

Myocardial Infarction, Ischaemic heart diseases, Coronary thrombosis, all pains in cardiac region.

ARTAV NADI AND HRIDAYA, NABHI, VASTI & GUD MARM (Ren channel - Extra channel)

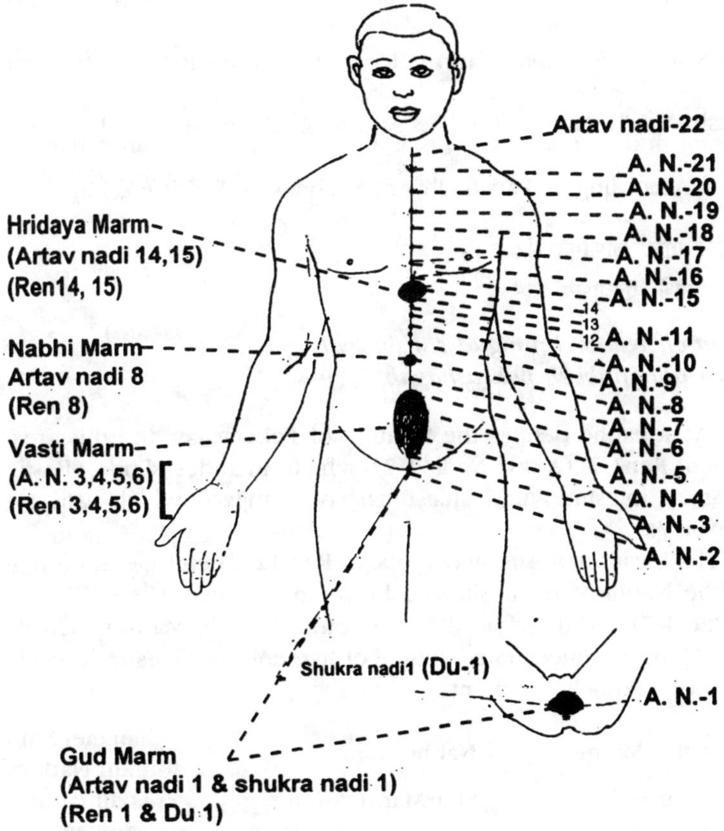

6 Pittaj and raktaj sira of udar (Abdomen) S. Sh. 7/7

Figure 35

Nabhi Marm (Figure 36)

पक्वामाशयोर्मध्ये सिराप्रभवा नाभिः, तत्रापि सद्योमरणम्।

(सु०शा०, 6/25)

Pakvamashayormadhye siraprabhava Nabhih,
Tatrapi Sadyomaranam

(Su. Sharir, 6/25)

According to S.Sh. 6/25, Nabhi Marm is located between Pakwashay and Amashaya.

To establish Nabhi Marm, it is necessary to define Pakwashay and Amashaya.

Pakwashay: According to Parishadhyam Shabdartha Sharirum, page 52.

तत समासेन वातः श्रोणीगुद संश्रयः।
तदुपरि अधोनाभेः पक्वाशयः

Tat samasen vatah shronigud sanshrayah
Tadupari adhonabheh pakvashayah

The word Adhonabhe defines the location of Pakwashay and this area comes between Ren1-7 (Artav Nadi 1-7) which includes Guda, Basti, Laghvantra (small intestine) and shleshmashay (Sanjiao) which are the principal seat of Vat.

Amashay: The location of Amashay is above Ren 12. Therefore according to definition the Nabhi Marm is situated between Amashay (Ren 12) and Pakwashay (Ren 1-7) and therefore the true point of Nabhi Marm is Ren 8.

This Nabhi Marm is concentrated source of live energy (lines of forces). This point is Judo's knock out point.

1.	Name of the Marm	Nabhi Marm
2.	Type of Marm	Sira Marm
3.	Prognosis	Sadya pranhar (sudden death)
4.	Quality Somya/Agneya	Agneya
5.	Size	*Svapanital kunchit sammit* 2.0 inches in diameter
6.	Location	Points Artav nadi 8 (Ren8)
7.	Indications	Apoplexy

Due to concentration of live forces it becomes very sensitive to any external and internal injury causing intense pain, shock and death.

ARTAV NADI AND HRIDAYA, NABHI, VASTI & GUD MARM (Ren channel - Extra channel)

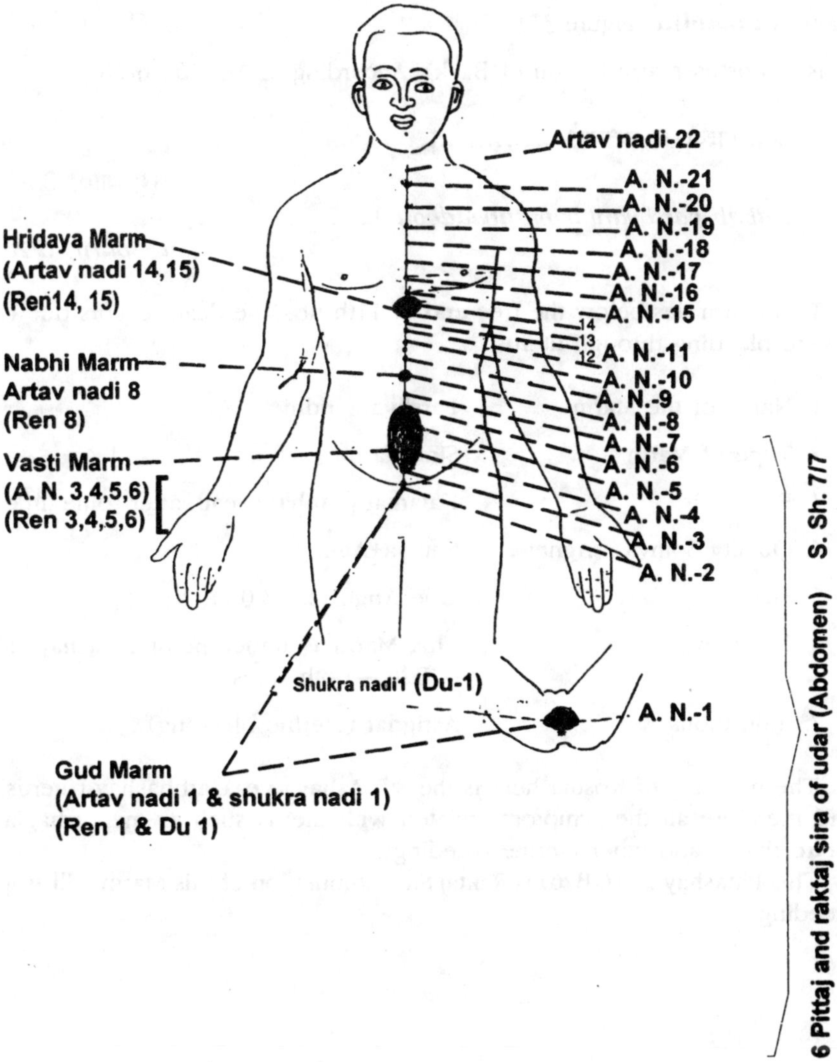

Figure 36

According to *Su.Sh.*, 7/36, damage to Sadyapranhar Marmas destroys the function of five sense organs and upsets reasoning leading to hallucination type symptoms causing intense and acute pain leading to shock.

We can resuscitate the patient by stimulating this Marm immediately after the shock. Siravedhan (acupuncture) is contra-indicated. For stimulation of this Marm only Agnikarm (Moxibustion) is permitted.

Parshva Sandhi (Figure 37)

This is Pristha Marm (Marm of Back). According to *Su. Sh.*, 6/26

अधः पार्श्वान्तर प्रतिबद्धौ ....

(सु०शा०, 6/26)

Aḍhah parshvantar pratibaddhou............

(Su. Sharir, 6/26)

This marm lies below the free end of 11th rib. The death occurs due to severe bleeding through uterus.

1. Name of the Marm	Parshva Sandhi
2. Type of Marm	Sira Marm
3. Prognosis	Kalantar pranhar (death after some time)
4. Quality Somya / Agneya :	Somya+Agneya
5. Size	One Angul 2.0–3.0 cm
6. Location	This Marm is under point Pittashay 26 (GB26)—both sides
7. Indications	Asrigdar (uterine bleeding)

The meaning of Kostha here is the 8th Ashaya i.e. Garbhashay (uterus) and therefore all the symptoms related with uterus such as menorrhagia, metrorrhagia and other uterine bleedings.

This Pittashay 26 (GB26) is Raktaj Sira, stimulation of this Marm will stop bleeding.

MARM AND VATAJ, PITTAJ, KAPHAJ AND RAKTAJ SIRAS OF PRISHTHA (BACK)

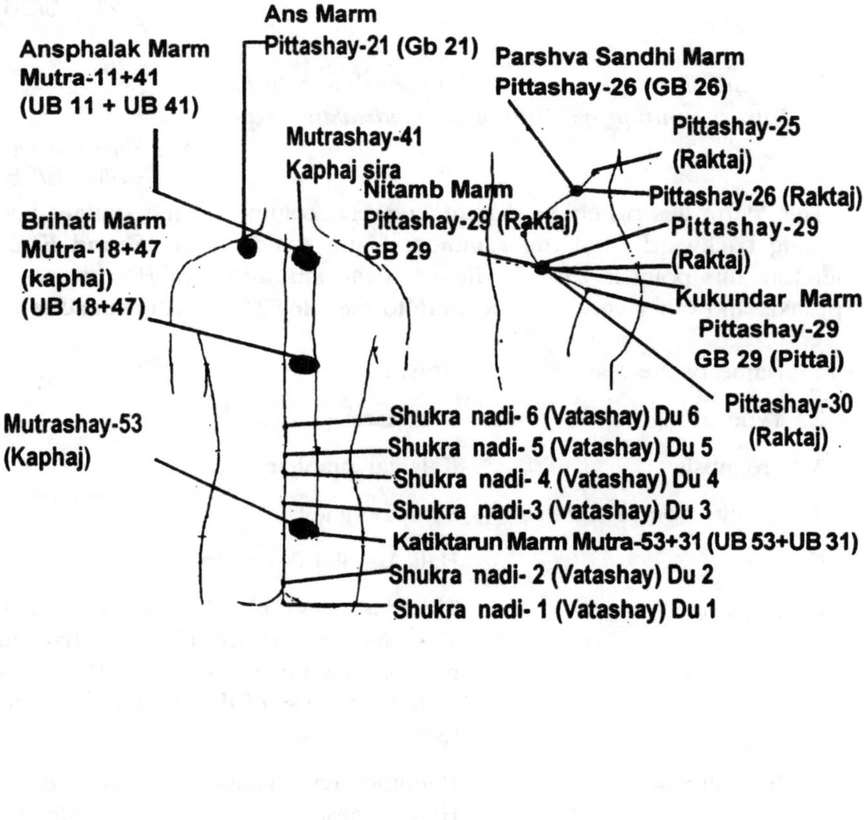

Figure 37

Brihati Marm (Figure 38)

This is also Prishtha Marm. According to *Su. Sharir,* 6/26

स्तनमूलादृजूभयतःपृष्ठवंशस्य बृहती
तत्रशोणितातिप्रवृत्तिनिमित्तैरूपद्रवैम्रियते।

(सु०शा०, 6/26)

Stanmooladrijoobhayatahprishthvanshasya brihati
Tatrashonitatipravrittinimittairupadravaimriyate.

(Su. Sharir, 6/26)

This Marm lies on either side of Vertebral column on the straight line running backward from the stanmool Marm which is St 18 and K 22 therefore this point is UB 18 which has the indications of Hematemesis, Epistaxis and other conditions leading to bleeding *(Shonitati pravritti)*

1. Name of the Marm	Brihati
2. Type of Marm	Sira Marm
3. Prognosis	Kalantar pranhar
4. Quality Somya/Agneya	Somya+Agneya
5. Size	Half Angul 1.0–1.5 cm
6. Location	This Marm lies under the point Mutrashay 47 + Mutrashay 18 UB 47+UB 18 (two in number) Two inches lateral to the tip of spinous process of the 9th thoracic vertebra.
7. Indications	Haemorrhagic disorders Hematemesis Epistaxis

MARM AND VATAJ, PITTAJ, KAPHAJ AND RAKTAJ SIRAS OF PRISHTHA (BACK)

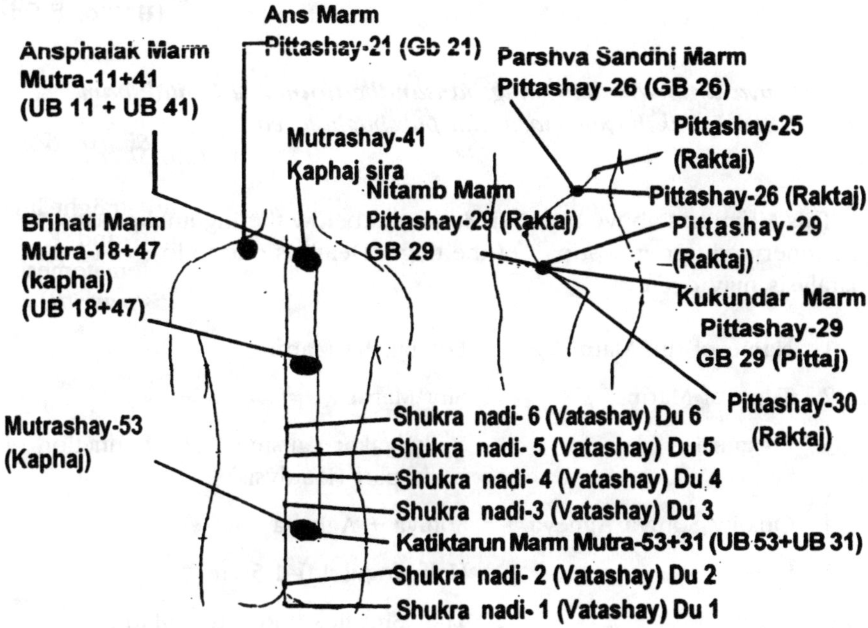

Figure 38

Lohitaksha Marm (Figure 39 A, 39 B)

This is also Sira Marm. This is Sakthi Marm (lies in extremities)

उर्व्या ऊर्ध्वमधो वङ्क्षणसंधेरुरुमूले लोहिताक्षं
तत्र लोहितक्षयेण मरणं पक्षाघातो वा।

(सु०शा०, 6/24)

Urvya urdhvamadho vangshansandherurumoole lohitaksham,
Tatra Lohitkshayen maranam pakshaghato va

(Su. Sharir, 6/24)

This Marm lies above the Urvi Marm and below the inguinal groove over the inner and uppermost part of the thigh. Death is due to loss of blood or paralysis may occur.

1.	Name of the Marm	Lohitaksha Marm
2.	Type of Marm	Sira Marm
3.	Prognosis	Vaikalyakar causing loss of function of body part (Paralysis)
4.	Quality Somya/Agneya	Somya + Agneya
5.	Size	Half Angul 1.0–1.5 cm
6.	Location	The Sira lies under this Marm : In lower extremity : Yakrit 11 (Liv 11) In upper extremity : Hridaya 1 (H 1). Centre of axilla, medial to axillary artery.
7.	Indications	Uterine bleeding Haemoptysis, Hemiplegia, Paraplegia.

Underneath this Marm lie branches of femoral artery and veins and branches of femoral nerve, therefore Sushrut has contra indicated Siravedhan (acupuncture) to prevent damage of above mentioned structures. AgniKarm (Moxibustion) is allowed.

LOHITAKSHA MARM, URDHVAGA HRIDAYA DHAMANI DHATU- PITTA AND RAKTA-STRI SANGYAK Ht.: Heart Channel (Yin)

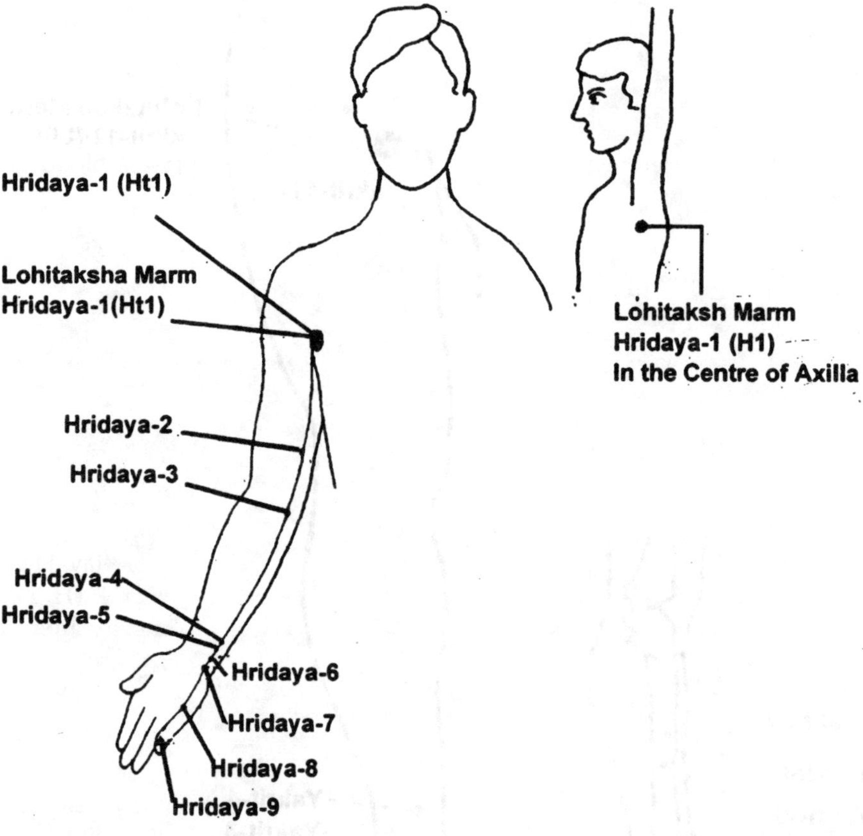

Figure 39 A

KSHIPRA MARM AND LOHITAKSHA MARM URDHVAGA YAKRIT DHAMANI- PITTA RAKTAJ (STRI SANGYAK- .YIN)

Liv : Liver Channel (Yin)

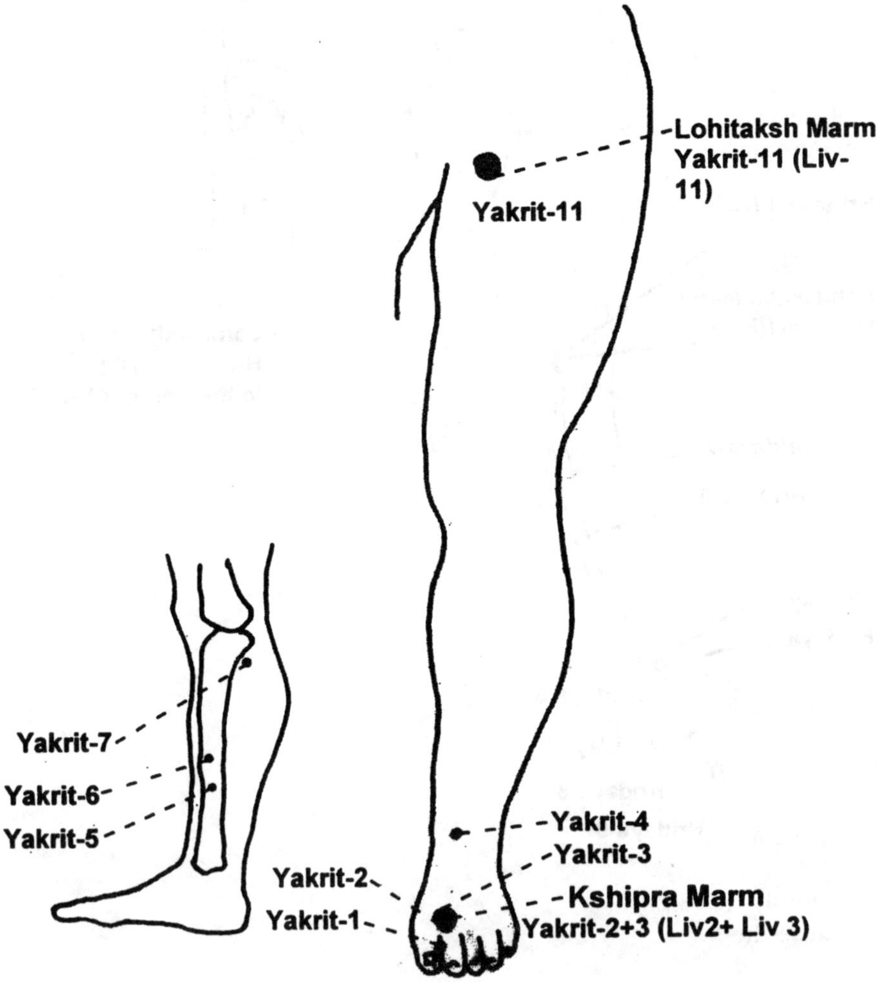

Figure 39 B

Urvi Marm (Figure 22, 40)
Urvi is Sakthi and Sira Marm.
(Marm of Extremity)

ऊरुमध्ये उर्वी तत्र शोणितक्षयात् सक्थिशोषः।

(सु०शा०, 6/24)

Urumadhye urvi tatra shonitkshayat sakthishoshah

(Su. Sharir, 6/24)

According to *Su. Sh.*, 6/24 this Marm lies in the centre of the thigh. Blood deficiency causes atrophy of muscles of the extremities. (see *Su. Sh.*, 15/9 for Atrophy of Muscles due to deficiency of blood).

1. Name of the Marm	Urvi
2. Type of Marm	Sira Marm
3. Prognosis	Vaikalyakar (Loss of function of any part of the body)
4. Quality Somya/Agneya	Somya + Agneya
5. Size	One Angul 2–3 cm
6. Location	The sira involved Amashay 32 and Mutrashay 37 (St 32 and UB 37). In lower extremity both have good efficacy. Talhridaya 2 (P2) in upper extremity
7. Indications	In lower extremity: Muscular atrophy, Motor impairment due to poor blood supply. In upper extremity: Cardiac Muscle Changes, Cardiac Pain.

According to *Su. Sh.*, 8/7 Siravedhan (acupuncture) is contraindicated for Urvi Marm. Agnikarm (Moxibustion) is allowed for the reasons given previously. For Urvi Marm both the points can be taken together or alone because their indications are same (Vaikalyakar - loss of function).

MARM AND ADHOGA AMASHAY DHAMANI PURUSH SANGYAK(YANG)
St : Stomach Channel (Yang)

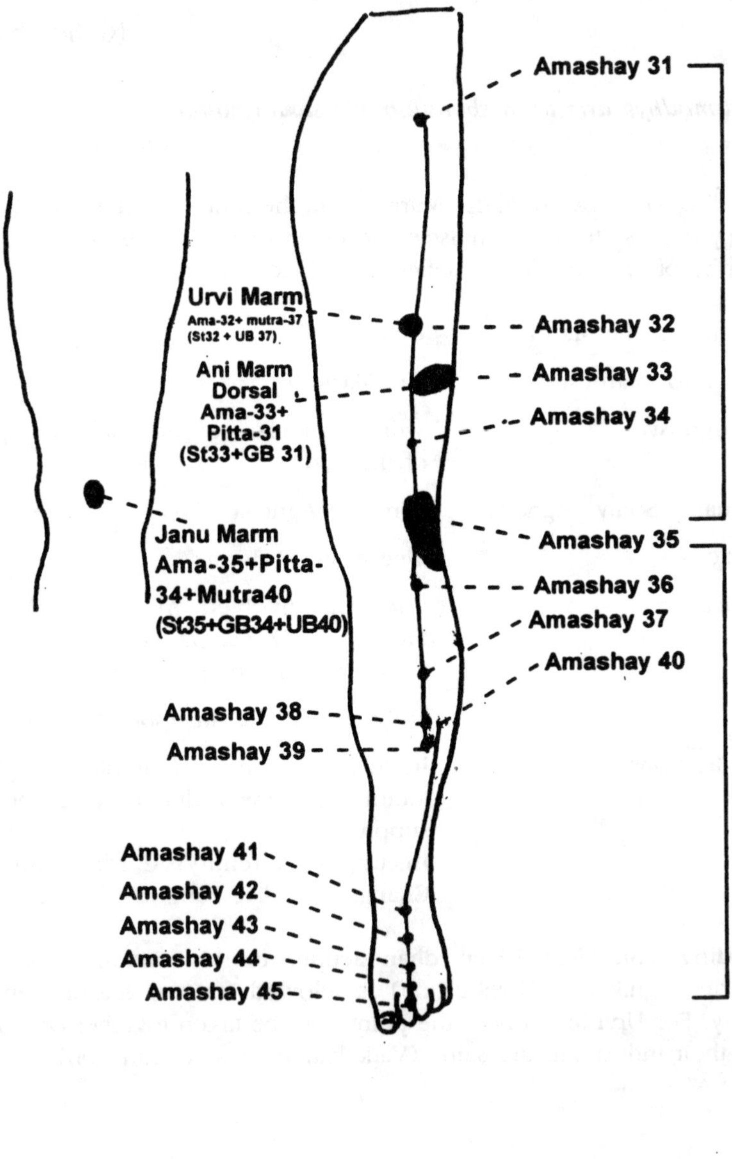

Figure 40

Snayu Marm

Snayu Marm are 27 in number. By Snayu we mean diseases of nervous system and alterations of nervous function including braincells, 12 cranial nerves, neurotransmitter and centres of different sense organs in the brain.

According to *Su. Nidan,* 1/29 when vayu is vitiated in Snayus it causes tremors, excruciating pain and spasmodic jerks and loss of motor and sensory functions.

Further in *Su. Sutra,* 25/37, he says when Snayus are afflicted patient becomes hunchback, the organs cannot perform their work and become devoid of their functions, with intense pain and healing of the disease becomes delayed.

The Snayu Marmas are following:

Ani Marma	-	4
Vitap Marma	-	2
Kakshadhar Marma	-	2
Kurch Marma	-	4
Kurchashir Marma	-	4
Vasti Marma	-	1
Kshipra Marma	-	4
Ansa Marma	-	2
Vidhur Marma	-	2
Utkshep Marma	-	2

Ani Marm (Figures 41, 42, 47)

These Marms lie in extremities and are of Snayu Marm variety. These are four in number. According to *Sushrut Sharir*, 6/24:

> जानुनऊर्ध्वमुभयतस्त्र्यङ्गुलमाणी तत्र
> शोफाभिवृद्धिः स्तब्धसक्थिता च।
>
> (सु०शा०, 6/24)

> *Janunurdhvamubhayatastrayangulamani tatra*
> *Shophabhivriddhih stabdhsakthita ch.*
>
> *(Su. Sharir, 6/24)*

Ani Marm lies on either side—3 fingers above the knee and elbow joints. Affliction of this Marm causes swelling of knee and elbow joint and numbness of the extremities.

1. Name of the Marm	Ani Marm
2. Type of Marm	Snayu Marm
3. Prognosis	Vaikalyakar (Loss of functions)
4. Somya/Agneya	Somya + Agneya
5. Size	1/2 Angul on each side, 1.0 cm – 1.5 cm
6. Location	Sirabindu Lower Extremity : Pittashay 31, Amashay 33 (Gb31 St33) *Adhah* (Yang) Yakrit 9, Pliha 10 (LIV 9, Sp10) *Urdhva* (Yin) Upper Extremity : Vrihadantra12, Shleshmashay11, Phuffus4 (LI12, Sj11, Lu4)
7. Indications	Hemiplegia, motor impairment

Ani Marm afflictions are diseases of nerves, cause is not local as in Janu Marm. Origin of both is different. In the disease named Krosthukshirsh these very points should be punctured for its cure. The same is in upper extremity.

MARM AND ADHOGA AMASHAY DHAMANI PURUSH SANGYAK(YANG)
St: Stomach Channel (Yang)

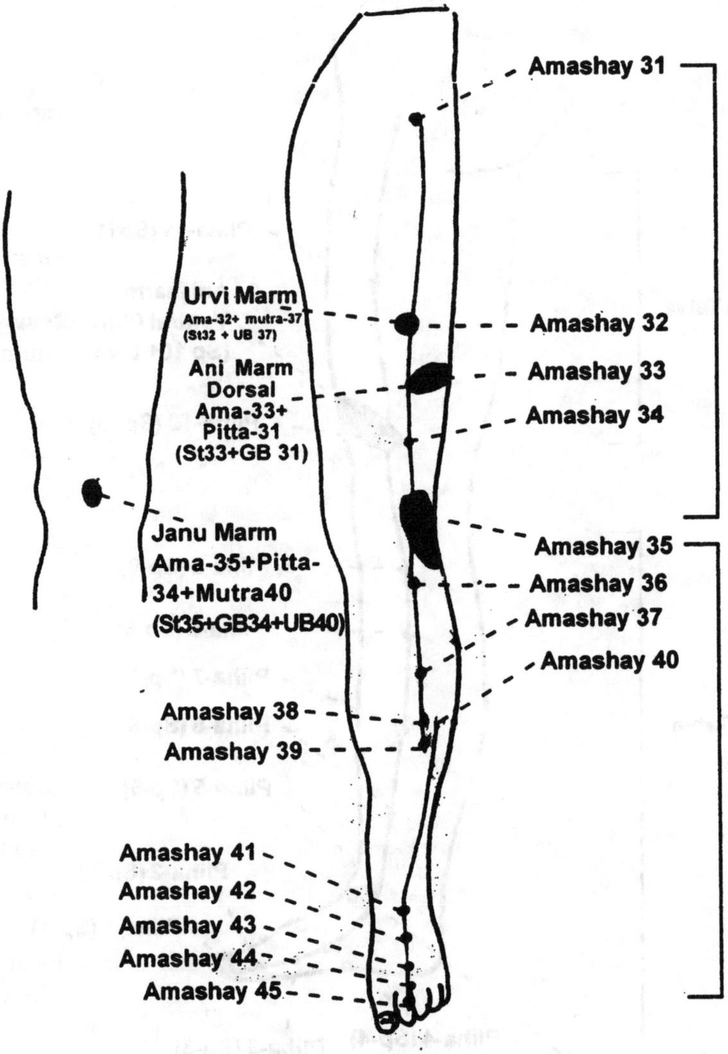

Figure 41

ANI MARM, KURCHSHIR MARM AND URDHVAGA PLIHA DHAMANI STRI SANGYAK (YIN)

Sp : Spleen Channel

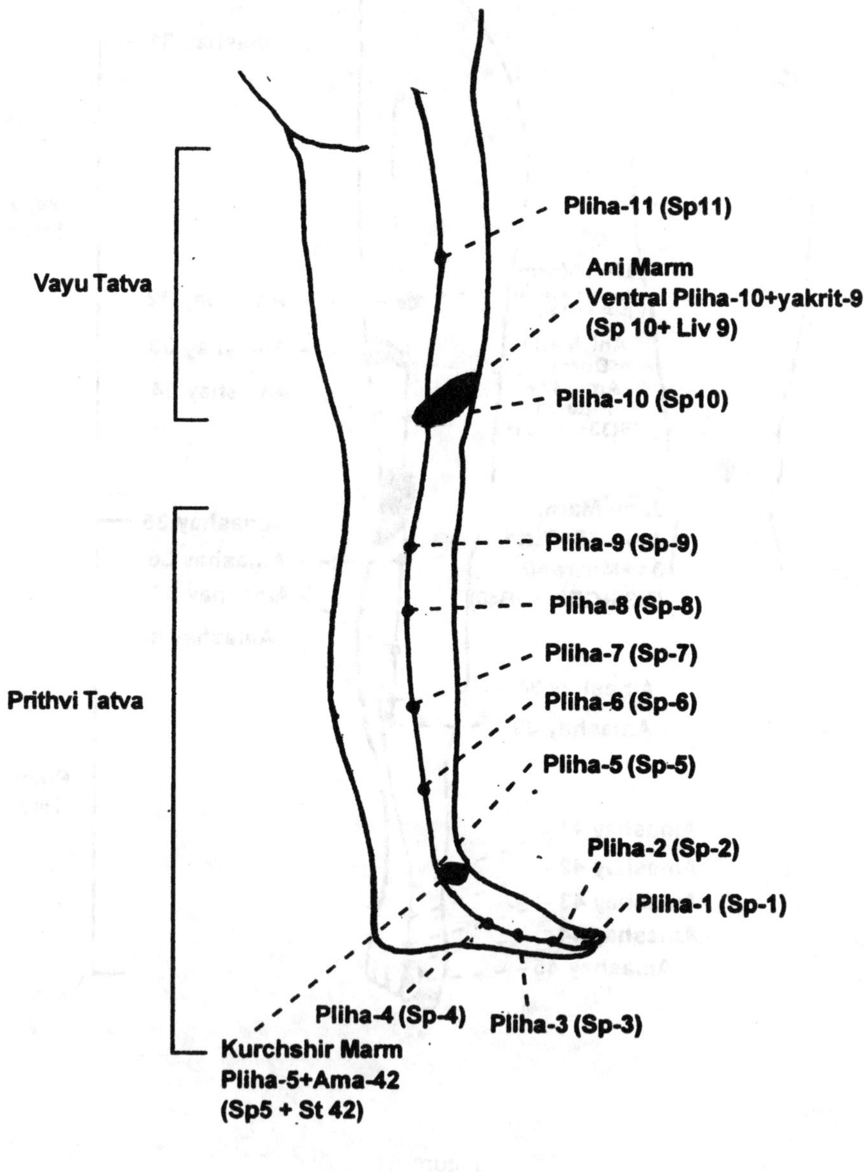

Figure 42

Vitap Marm (Figure, 43)

This is the Marm of upper part of the lower extremity and is of Snayu Marm variety.

According to *Su.Sh.*, 6/24:

वङ्क्षणवृषणयोरन्तरे विटपं
तत्र षाण्ढ्यमल्पशुक्रता वा भवति

(सु०शा०, 6/24)

Vankshanvrishanayorantare vitapam
Tatra shandhyamalpashukrata va bhavati

(Su. Sharir, 6/24)

The Vitap Marm lie in between the scrotum and inguinal canal, cause impotency and oligospermia (Sperm count less than 20 million).

1. Name of the Marm	Vitap Marm
2. Type of Marm	Snayu Marm
3. Prognosis	Vaikalyakar Marm (Loss of function)
4. Quality Somya / Agneya :	Somya + Agneya
5. Size	One Angul 2.0–3.0 cm
6. Location	Sirabindu Vrikka 11 (K11) on the superior border of symphysis pubis, half inch lateral to midline.
7. Indications	Impotency and Oligospermia related to C.N.S

This impotency and oligospermia is of central Nervous System origin as it is Snayu Marm variety because CNS modulates erectile response via pathways descending through the lateral column of the Spinal Cord.

URDHAVGA VRIKA DHAMANI, VITAP MARM AND KAPHAJ SIRAS OF KOSHTHA (TORSO) - STRI SANGYAK
K : Kidney Channel (Yin)

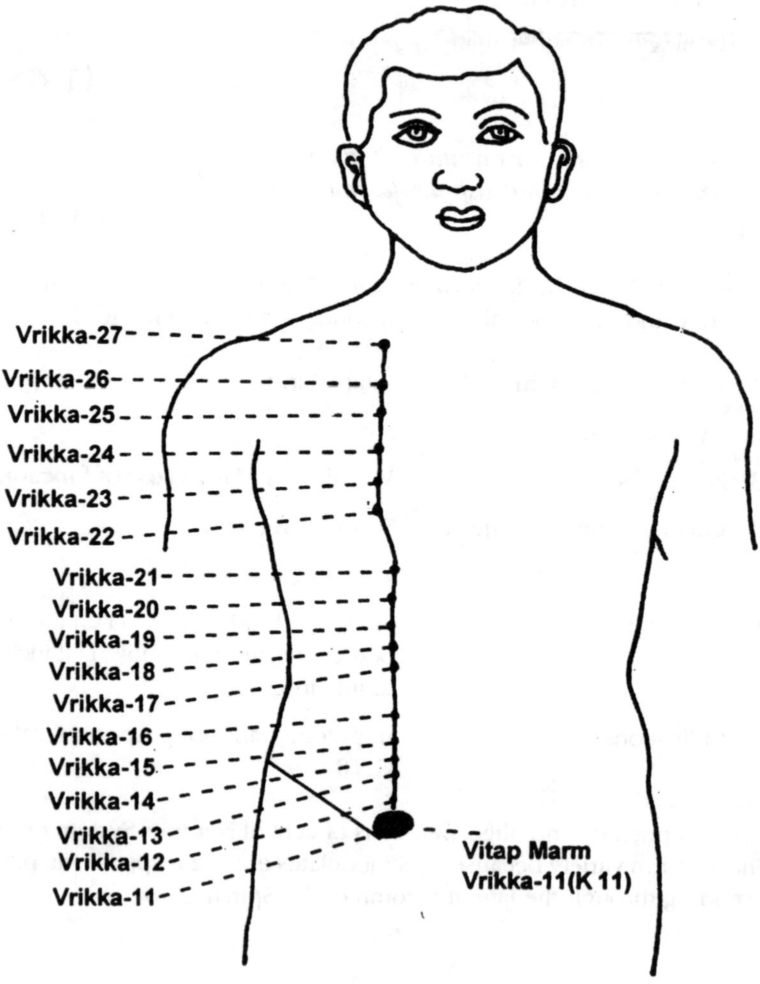

Figure 43

Kakshadhar Marm (Figure 44)

वक्षः कक्षयोर्मध्ये कक्षधरं
........कक्षधरे पक्षाघातः

(सु०शा०, 6/24)

Vakshah kakshyormadhye kakshadharam
..................*kakshadhare pakshaghatah*

(Su. Sharir, 6/24)

This is the Marm of upper extremity and is of Snayu Marm variety.

According to *Sushrut Sharir,* 6/24, this Marm lies in between chest and axillary pit. When Hemiplegia occurs this marm is damaged (due to involvement of underlying nerves, ulnar nerve, median nerve and branch of brachial cutaneous nerve).

1. Name of Marm	Kakshadhar
2. Type of Marm	Snayu Marm
3. Prognosis	Vaikalyakar
4. Somya/Agneya	Somya + Agneya
5. Size	Half Angul 1.0 cm –1.5 cm
6. Location	Sirabindu Shleshmashay 14 (Sj 14) between the acromion and greater tuberosity of humerus.
7. Indications	*Kakshdhare pakshaghatah (Su. Sharir, 6/24)* Hemiplegia and loss of function of arm. Method of Stimulation Sira vedhan 0.5-1.0" Agnikarm (Moxibustion can be done)

TIRYAGA SLESHMASHAY DHAMANI, MARM AND SIRAS PURUSH SANGYAK (YANG)

Sj: Sanjiao Channel (Yang)

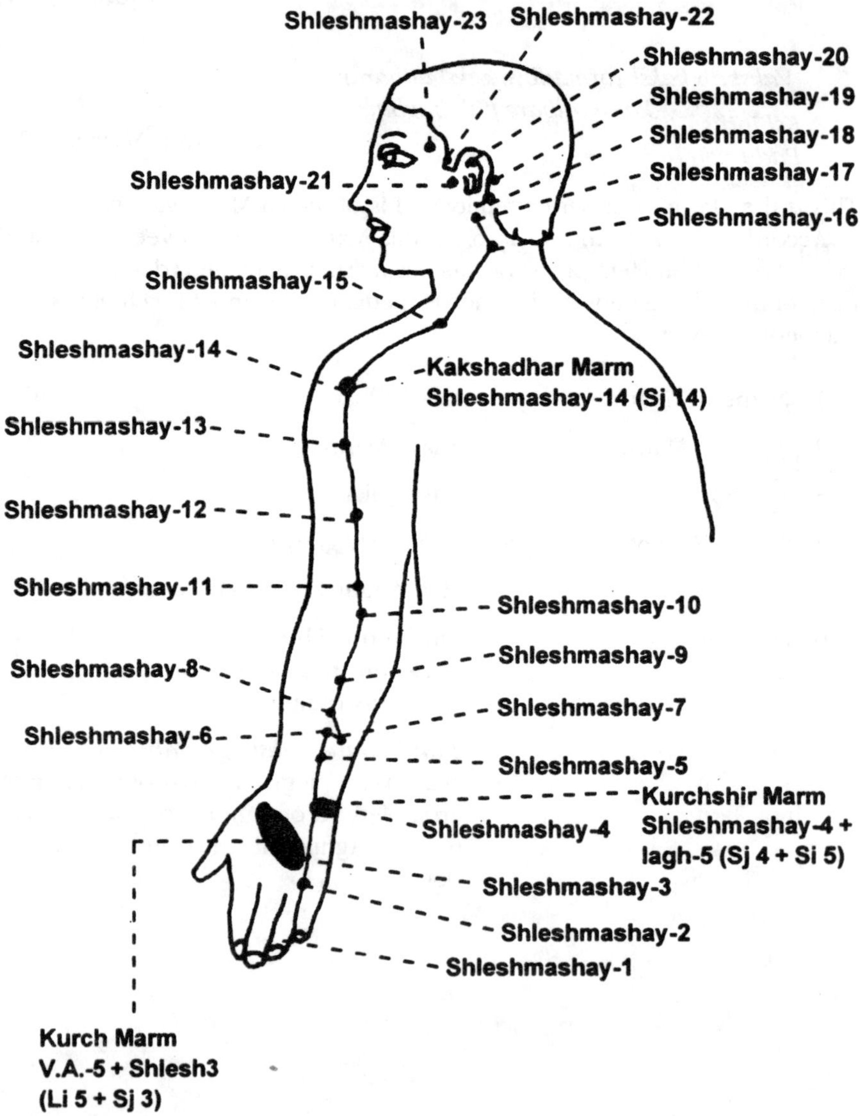

Figure 44

Kurch Marm (Figures 45, 46, 47)

These are the Marmas of extremities and are of Snayu Marm variety and total four in number. According to *Su.Sh.*, 6/24:

क्षिप्रस्योपरिष्टादुभयतः कूर्चो नाम, तत्र पादस्य भ्रमणवेपने

(सु०शा०, 6/24)

Kshiprasyoparishtadubhayatah kurcho nam, Tatra Padasya bhramanvepane

(Su. Sharir, 6/24)

This marm lies on the foot and hand just above the Kshipra Marm on both sides.

1. Name of the Marm	Kurch Marm
2. Type of Marm	Snayu Marm
3. Prognosis	Vaikalyakar
4. Quality Somya/Agneya	Somya + Agneya
5. Size	*Svapanital kunchit sammit* (2" in diameter)
6. Location	Sirabindu Upper Extremity : Vrihadantra$_5$, Shleshmashay 3 LI 5, SJ 3. Lower Extremity : Pittashay 42, yakrit 3 GB42 LIV3.
7. Indications	Pain and Motor impairment of hand and leg. Both of these lie on the dorsum of foot and hand. Method of Stimulation is Siravedhan and AgniKarm. (Moxibustion)

KURCH MARM, GULPH MARM AND PITTASHAY DHAMANI OF SAKTHI, PURUSH SANGYAK (YANG) & Gb: Gall-bladder Channel

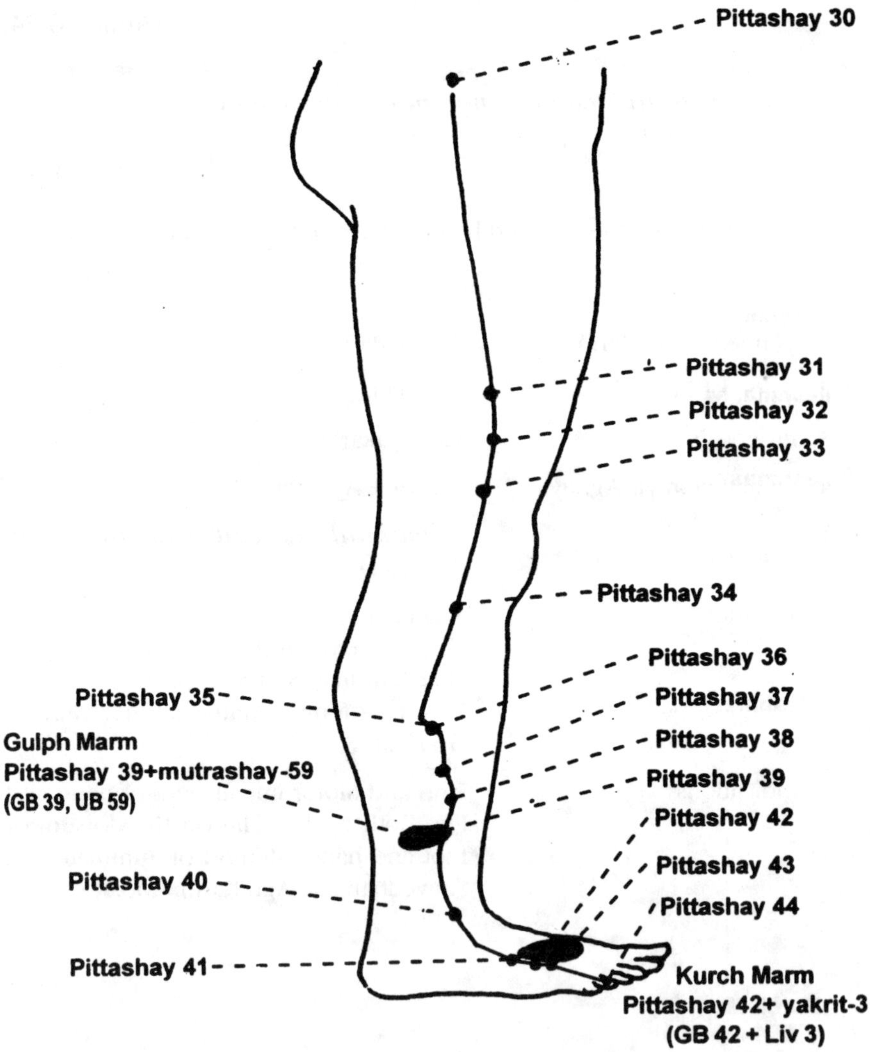

Figure 45

TIRYAGA SHLESHMASHAY DHAMANI, MARM AND SIRAS PURUSH SANGYAK (YANG)

Sj : Sanjiao Channel (Yang)

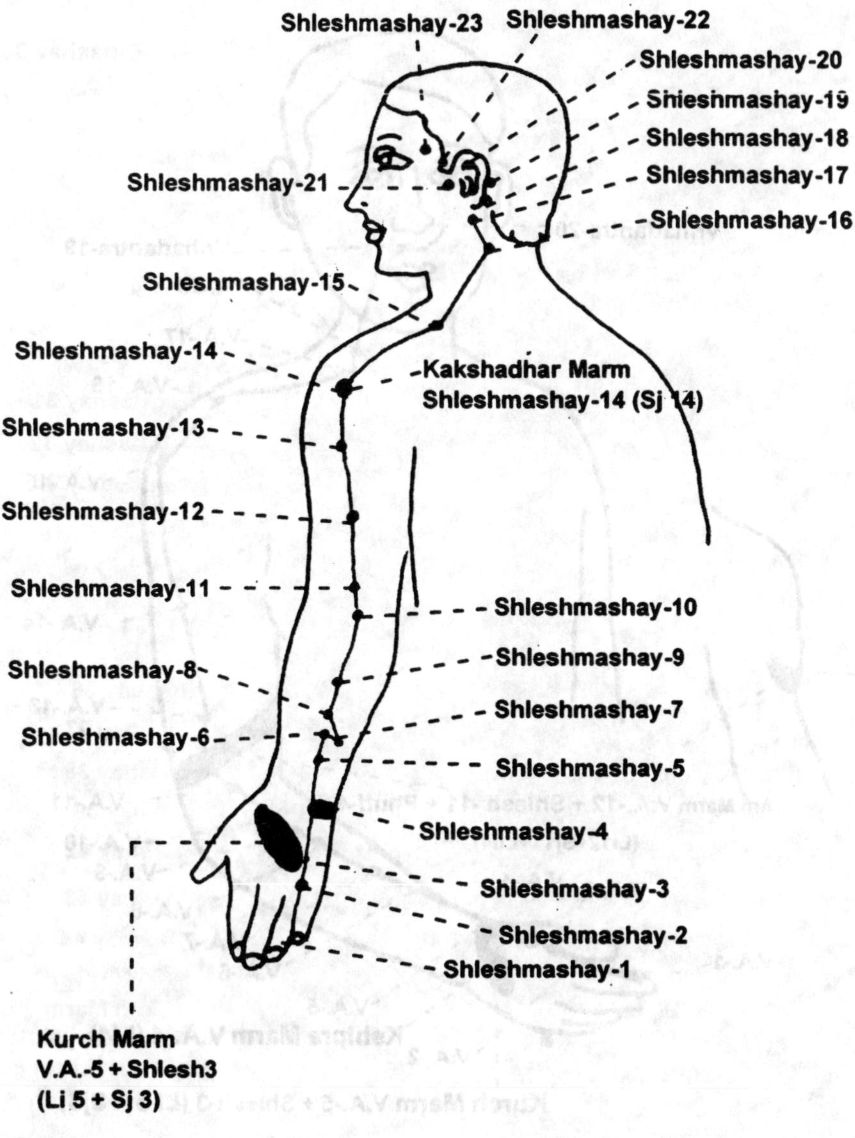

Figure 46

ADHOGA VRIHADANTRA DHAMANI (VATASHAY-APAN VAYU) & VATAJ SIRAS-PURUSH SANGYAK (Yang)
Li: Large intestine channel

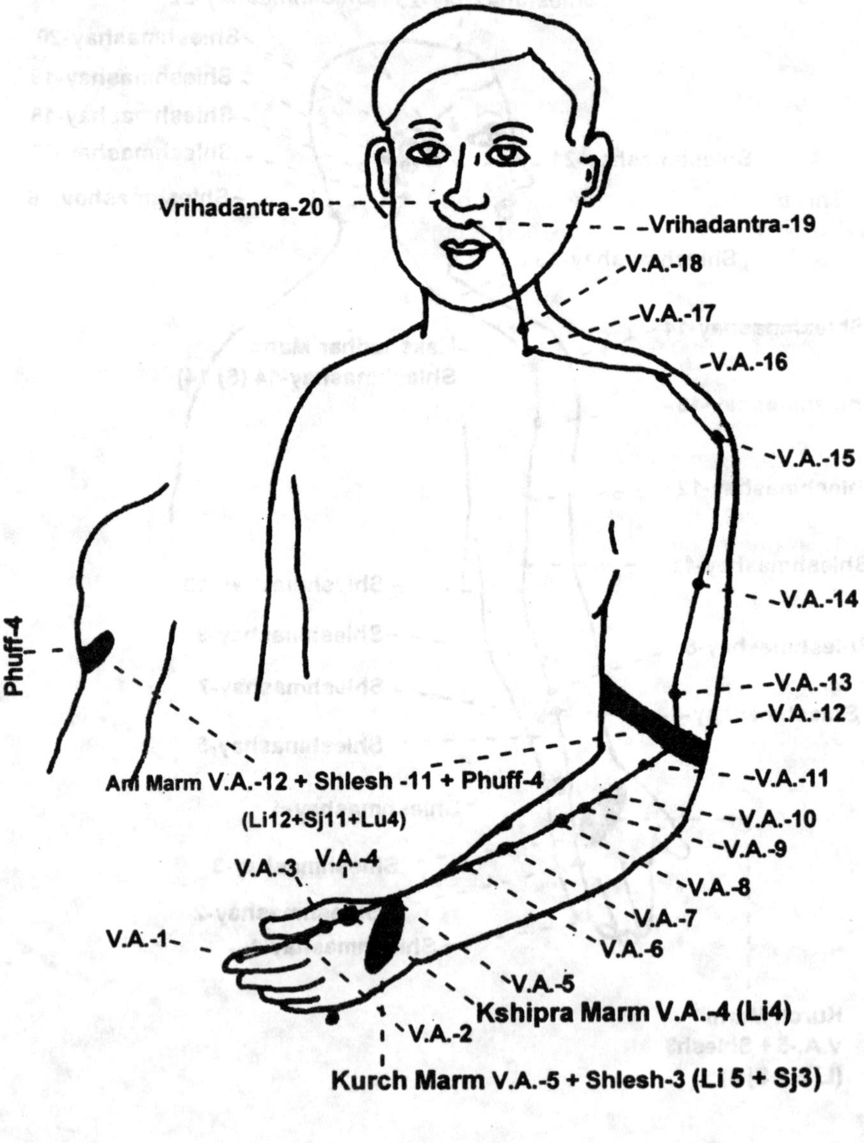

Figure 47

Kurchashir Marm (Figure 48, 49)

These are also the Marm of extremities and are four in number and are of Snayu Marm variety. According to *Su.Sh.*, 6/24:

गुल्फसन्धेरध उभयतः कूर्चशिरः तत्र रुजाशोफौ।

(सु०शा०, 6/24)

Gulphsandheradh ubhayatah kurchshiràh tatra rujashophou

(Su. Sharir, 6/24)

This marm lies just below the Gulph Marm on either side. When this Marm is diseased pain and inflammation occurs.

According to *Sushrut Nidan, 1/27:*

स्नायुप्राप्तः स्तम्भकम्पौ शूलमाक्षेपणं तथा।

(सु०नि०, 1/27)

Snayupraptah stambhkampou shulmakshepanam tatha

(Su. Nidan, 1/27)

1. Name of the Marm	Kurchashir
2. Type of Marm	Snayu Marm
3. Prognosis	Rujakar Marm
4. Quality Somya /Agneya	Agni + Vayu
5. Size	One angul (2.0–3.0 cm)
6. Location	Sirabindu Lower Extremity : Pliha 5, Amashay 42 (Sp5, St42) Upper Extremity : Shleshmashay 4, Laghvantra 5 (Sj4, Si5)
7. Indications	Pain and inflammation on the dorsum of hand and foot.

TIRYAGA SHLESHMASHAY DHAMANI, MARM AND SIRAS PURUSH SANGYAK (YANG)

Sj: Sanjiao Channel (Yang)

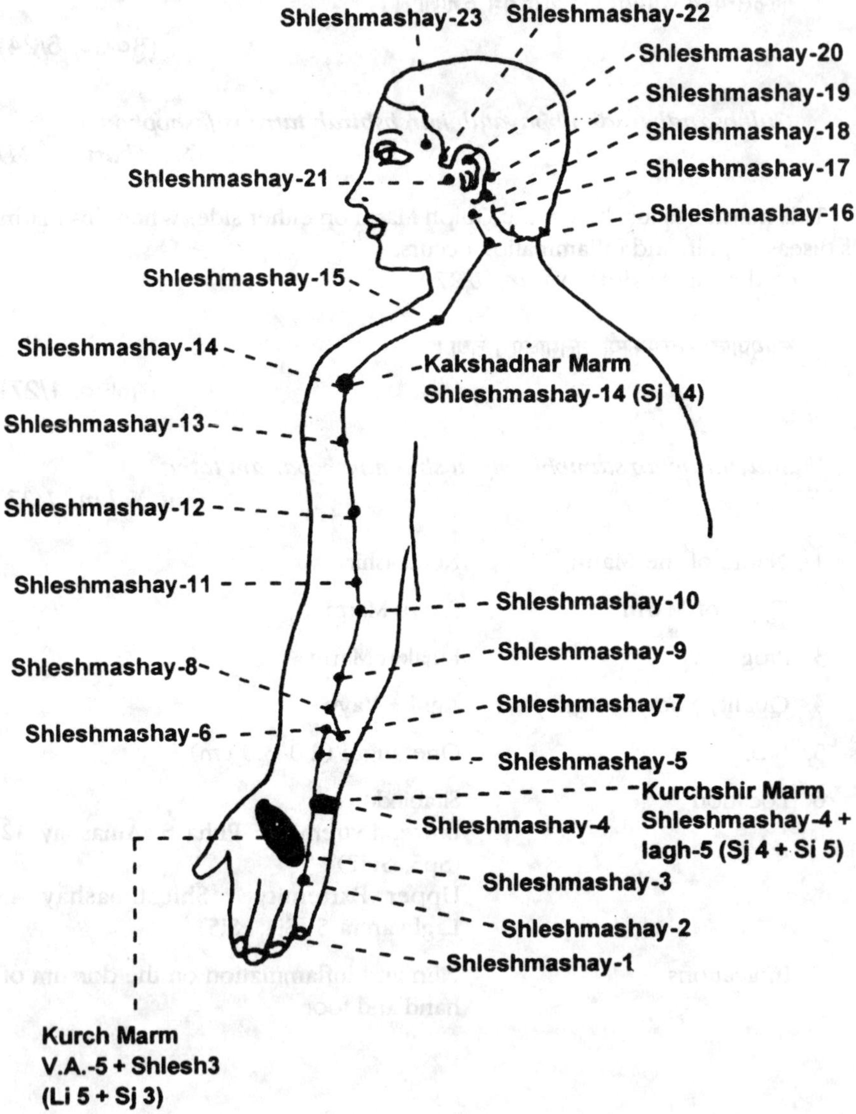

Figure 48

ANI MARM, KURCH SHIR MARM AND URDHVAGA PLIHA DHAMANI STRI SAṄGYAK (YIN)

Sp: Spleen Channel

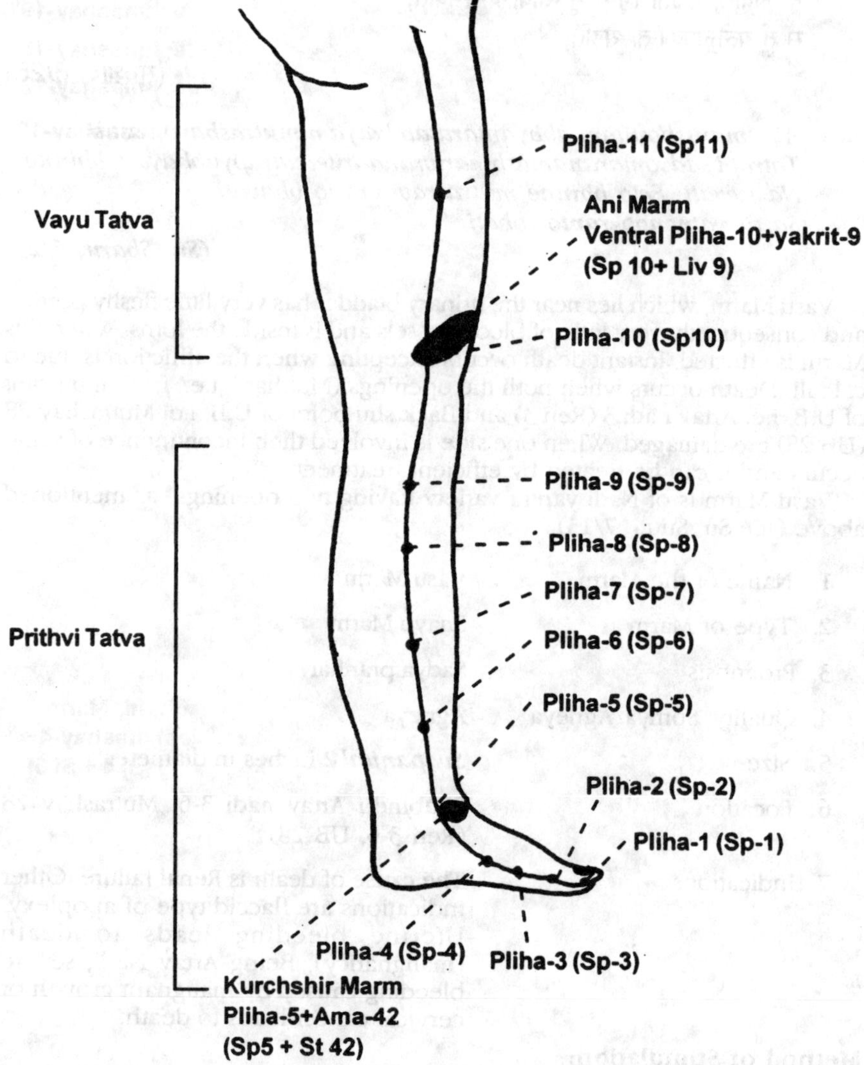

Figure 49

Vasti Marm (Figure 50)

This is the Marm of abdomen and is of Snayu Marm variety. One in number.

According to Su. Sharir 6/25:

अल्पमांसशोणितां ऽभ्यंतरतः कट्यां मूत्राशयो बस्तिः,
तत्रापि सद्योमरणमश्मरीव्रणादृते, तत्राप्युभयतो भिन्ने
न जीवति, एकतो भिन्ने मूत्रस्रावी व्रणोभवति,
स तुं यत्नेनोपक्रान्तो रोहति;

(सु०शा०, 6/25)

Alpamansshonitam abhyantaratah katyam mutrashayo vastih,
Tatrapi sadyomaranamashmarivranadrite, tatrapyubhayato bhinne
Na jeevati, Ekto bhinne mutrasravi vrano bhavati,
Sa tu yatnenopkranto rohati.

(Su. Sharir, 6/25)

Vasti Marm, which lies near the urinary bladder has very little fleshy portion and consequently very little of blood vessels and is inside the loins. When this Marm is afflicted, instant death occurs excepting when the affliction is due to calculi. Death occurs when both the openings (Mukhani, i.e., front mu point of U.B. i.e. Artav nadi 3 (Ren 3) and Back shu point of U.B. i.e. Mutrashay 28 (UB 28) are damaged. When one side is involved then incontinence of urine occurs and it can be treated by efficient treatment.

Vasti Marm is of Nadi yantra variety having two openings as mentioned above (see Su. Sutra, 7/13).

1. Name of the Marm	Vasti Marm
2. Type of Marm	Snayu Marm
3. Prognosis	Sadya pranhar
4. Quality: Somya/Agneya	Agneya
5. Size	*Svapanital* 2 inches in diameter
6. Location	Sirabindu Artav nadi 3-6, Mutrashay 28 (Ren 3-6, UB 28)
7. Indications	The cause of death is Renal failure. Other indications are flaccid type of apoplexy. Uterine bleeding leads to death (malignancy), Being Artav Nadi, severe bleeding caused by malignant growth or cervical cancer leads to death.

Method of Stimulation:

All the above said points should be pricked including Mutrashay 28 (UB 28) and then heat is to be applied to the needles to create Agnikarm (moxibustion) effect.

Siravedhan - 0.5 - 1.0" perpendicularly.

ARTAV NADI AND HRIDAYA, NABHI, VASTI AND GUD MARM (Ren channel - Extra channel)

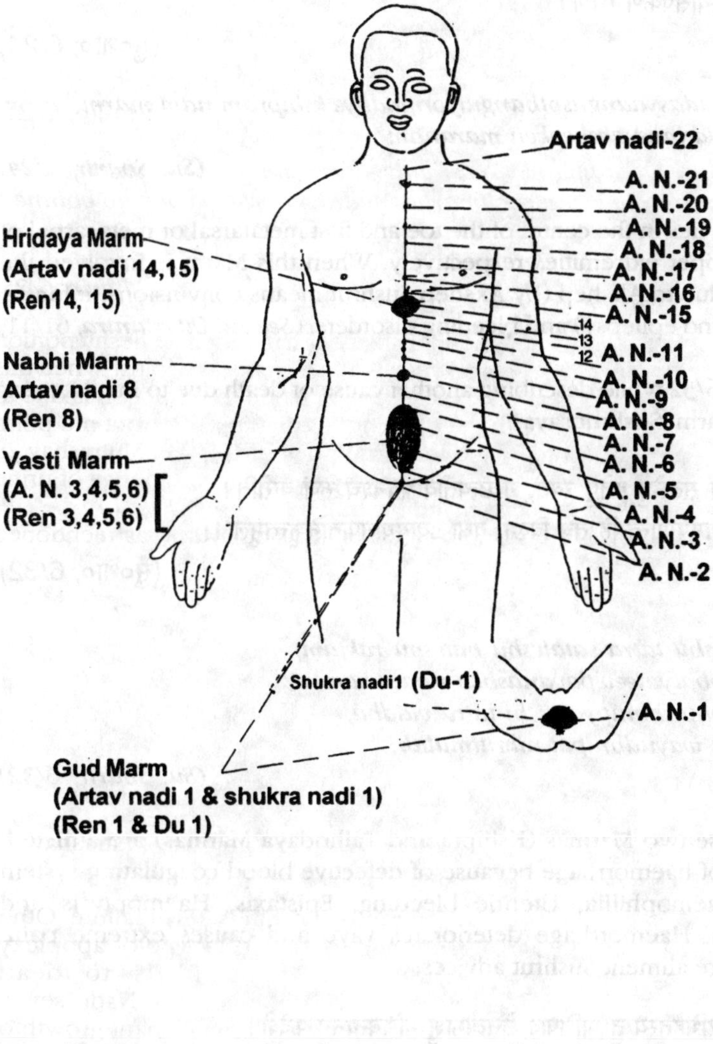

6 Pittaj and raktaj sira of udar (Abdomen) S. Sh. 7/7

Figure 50

Kshipra Marm (Figures 51, 52)

This is the Marm of extremities and is of Snayu Marm variety. According to *Su. Sh.*, 6/24:

तत्र पादस्याङ्गुष्ठाङ्गुल्योर्मध्ये क्षिप्रं नाम मर्म,
तत्र विद्धस्याक्षेपकेण मरणं।

(सु०शा०, 6/24)

Tatra padasyaangushthangulyormadhye kshipram nam marm
Tatra viddhasyakshepken maranam

(Su. Sharir, 6/24)

This Marm lies in the centre of the toe and first metatarsal or metacarpal of lower and upper extremities respectively. When this Marm is involved the patient dies due to Akshep (by Akshep Sushrut means convulsions, infantile convulsions and epilepsy) and bleeding disorders. (*See Su. Uttartantra,* 61/11, 12,13).

In *Su.Sh.*, 6/32 while describing another cause of death due to involvement of Kshipra Marm, Sushrut says:

क्षिप्रेषु तत्र सतलेषु हतेषु रक्तं, गच्छत्यतीव पवनश्च रुजं करोति।
एवं विनाशमुपयान्ति हि तत्र विद्धा, वृक्षा इवायुधनिपातनिकृत्तमूला।।

(सु०शा०, 6/32)

Kshipreshu tatra sataleshu hateshu raktam,
Gachchhatyateev pavanashch rujam karoti.
Evam vinashmupyanti hi tatra viddha,
Vriksha ivayudhnipat nikrittmulah.

(Su. Sharir, 6/32)

When these two Marmas (Kshipra and Talhridaya Marmas) are afflicted, patient dies of haemorrhage because of defective blood coagulating system including Haemophillia, Uterine bleeding, Epistaxis, Haemoptysis and Hemetemesis. Haemorrhage deteriorates vayu and causes extreme pain. Further to cure ailment Sushrut advices:

तस्मात्तयोरभिहतस्य तु पाणिपादं छेत्तव्यमाशु मणिबन्धनगुल्फदेशे।

(सु०शा०, 6/33)

Tasmattayorabhihatasya tu panipadam chettavyamashu manibandhangulphdeshe.

(Su. Sharir, 6/33)

We must stop bleeding by chedan (Siravedhan - acupuncture and moxibution) of the siras (points) near about Maniband and Gulpha area including both kshipra Marmas. Gulpha Pradesh (gulph area - siras of extremities near ankle joint).

Lower Extremity:

Vrikka3, 4, 6 (K, 3, 4, 6)	- For Haemoptysis (stops bleeding by the action of Himkriya)
Mutrashay58, 60 (UB 58, 60)	- For Epistaxis (stops bleeding by the action of Himkriya)
Phiha6 (Sp 6)	- For irregular menstruation and uterine bleeding. (stops bleeding by the action of Bhasm Avachurnan).
Yakrit2, 3, 5 (Liv2, 3, 5,)	- For irregular menstruation and uterine bleeding (stops bleeding by Dagdh kriya)

Manibandh Pradesh

Laghvantra 3 (SI 3)	- For Epistaxis (stops bleeding by dagdhakriya-(cauterization).
Talhridaya 4 (P 4)	- For Epistaxis, Hematemesis
Phuffus9, 10 (Lu 9, 10)	- For Haemoptyis (stops bleeding by Kashay-Astringent action)
Vrihadantra4 (LI 4)	- For Epistaxis and other coagulating defects. (stops bleeding by Kashay-Astringent action)

1. Name of the Marm	Kshipra Marm
2. Type of Marm	Snayu Marm
3. Prognosis	Kalantar Pranhar
4. Quality Somya/Agneya	Somya + Agneya
5. Size	Half Angul (1.0–1.5 cm)
6. Location	Sirabindu *Upper extremity:* Vrihadantra4 (LI 4) between first and Second Metacarpal bones. *Lower Extremity:* Yakrit 2, 3 (Liv - 2,3) situated in between first and second metatarsal bones.
7. Indications	Pain, bleeding disorders and Convulsions.

URDHVAGA YAKRIT DHAMANI, PITTA- RAKTAJ (STRI SANGYAK) KSHIPRA MARM AND LOHITAKSHA MARM Liv : Liver Channel (Yin)

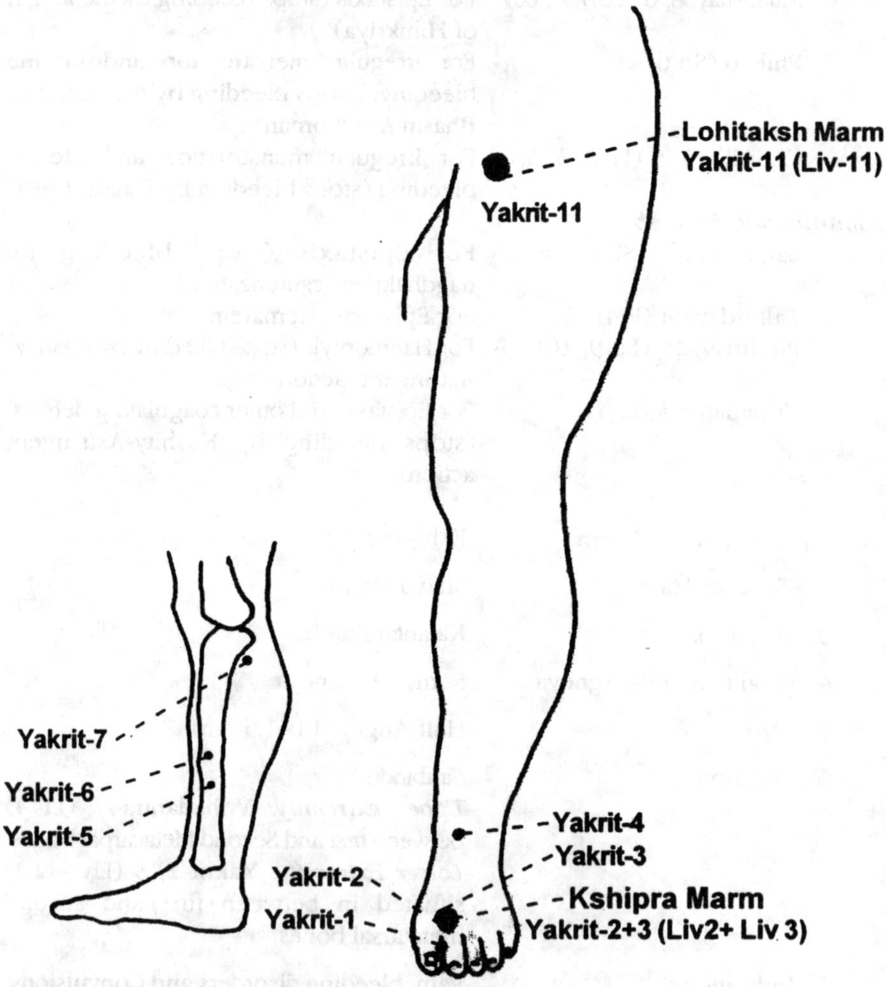

Figure 51

ADHOGA VRIHADANTRA DHAMANI (VATASHAY-APAN VAYU) & VATAJ SIRAS-PURUSH SANGYAK (Yang)
Li: Large intestine channel

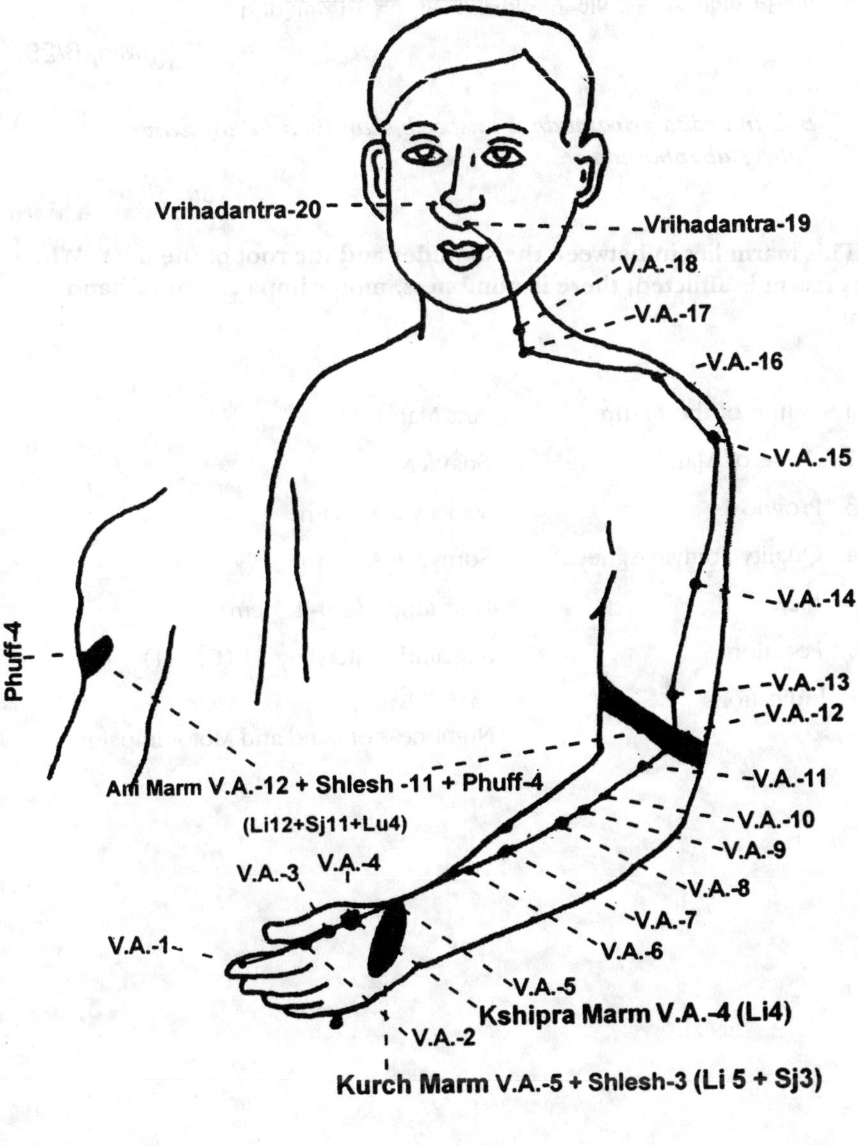

Figure 52

Ans Marm (Figure 53)

This is Prishtha Marm (on the back) and is of Snayu Marm variety. According to *Su. Sharir,* 6/26:

बाहुमूर्ध ग्रीवामध्ये अंस पीठ स्कन्धबन्धनावंसौ, तत्र स्तब्धबाहुता ।

(सु०शा०, 6/26)

Bahumurdha grivamadhye anspeeth skandhbandhanavanso,
Tatra stabdhbahuta.

(Su. Sharir, 6/26)

This marm lies in between the shoulder and the root of the neck. When this marm is afflicted, there is numbness, motor impairment of hand and arm.

1. Name of the Marm	Ans Marm
2. Type of Marm	Snayu Marm
3. Prognosis	Vaikalyakar Marm
4. Quality Somya/Agneya	Somya + Agneya
5. Size	Half angul (1.0–1.5 cm)
6. Location	Sirabindu Pittashay 21 (GB 21)
7. Indications	*Stabdhbahuta* Numbness of hand and Motor impairment.

MARM AND VATAJ, PITTAJ, KAPHAJ AND RAKTAJ SIRAS OF PRISHTHA (BACK)

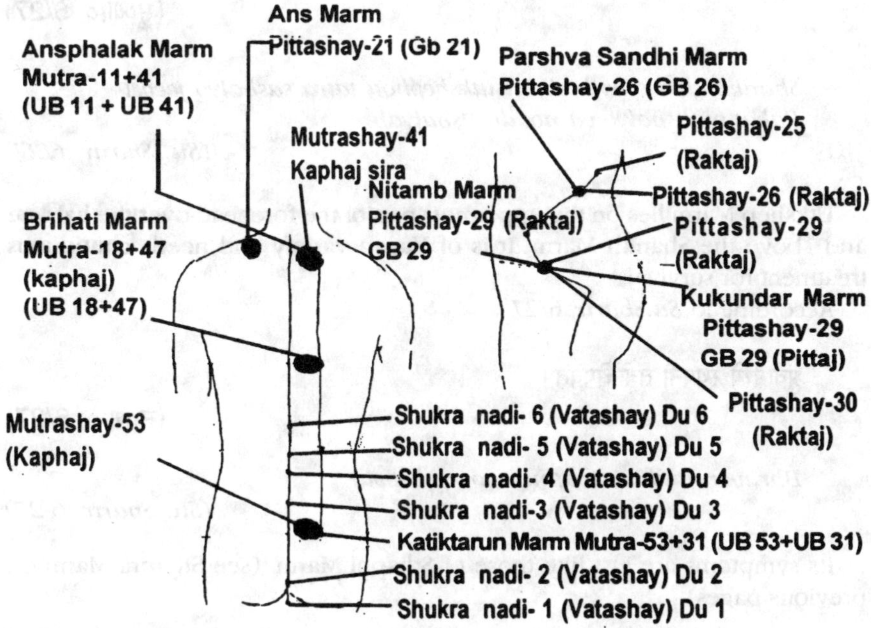

Figure 53

Utkshep Marm (Figure 54)

Utkshep is a Snayu Marm of head. According to *Su.Sharir*, 6/27:

शंखयोरूपरि केशान्त उत्क्षेपौ, तत्र सशल्यो जीवेत् पाकात्
पतितशल्यो वा नोद्धृतशल्यः।

(सु०शा०, 6/27)

Shankhayorupari keshant utkshephou tatra sashalyo jeevet
Pakat patitshalyo va noddhritshalyah.

(Su. Sharir, 6/27)

Utkshep Marm lies on the uppermost part of the forehead over the hairline and above the Shankh Marm. It is of Yapya variety and needs continuous treatment for survival.

According to *Su.Sharir*, 6/27:

भ्रुवोर्मध्ये स्थपनी तत्रोत्क्षेपवत्।

(सु०शा०, 6/27)

Bhruvormadhye sthapni, tatrotkshepvat

(Su. Sharir, 6/27)

Its symptoms are just like those of Sthapni Marm. (see Sthapni Marm on previous pages).

1. Name of the Marm	Utkshep Marm
2. Type of Marm	Snayu Marm
3. Prognosis	Vishalyaghn (needs continuous treatment)
4. Quality Somya/Agneya	Vayavya
5. Size	Half angul (1.0 cm –1.5 cm)
6. Location	Given above. By the side of Amashay 8 (St 8). It is an extra channel.
7. Indications	Infantile Convulsions Epilepsy, Mental disorder, Vertigo (central - not cochlear).

MARM, PITTAVAHINI DHAMANI AND SIRA OF URDHVAJATRU (ABOVE CLAVICLE)

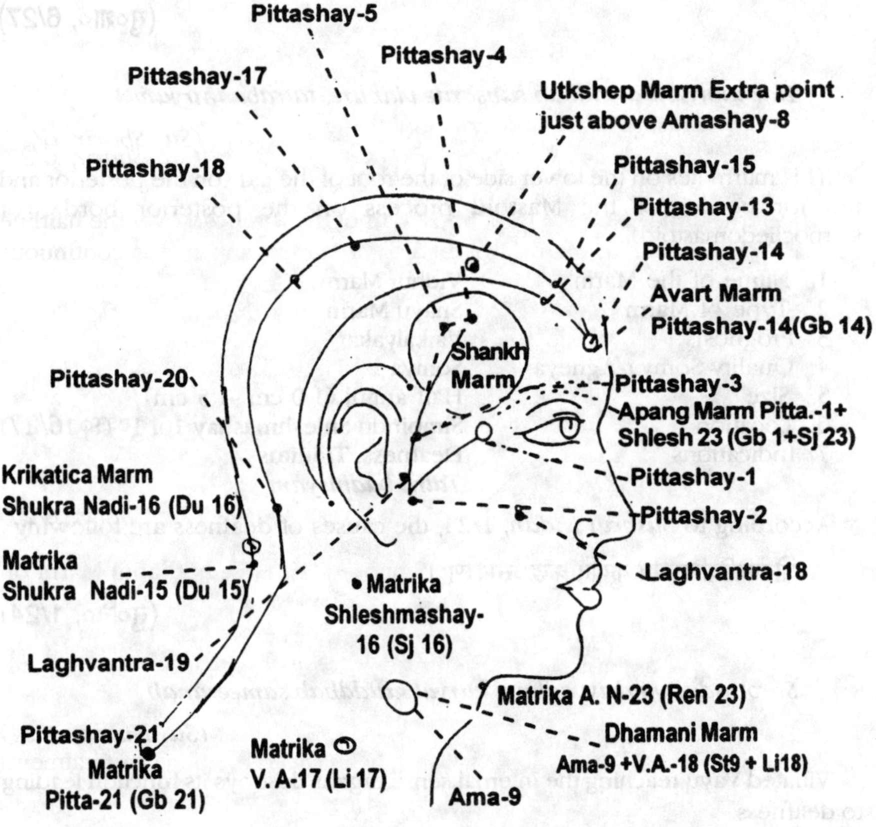

Figure 54

Vidhur Marm (Figure 55)

This is Urdhvajatru Marm (marm above the clavicle) and is of Snayu Marm variety.

According to *Su.Sharir*, 6/27:

कर्णपृष्ठतोऽधः संश्रिते विधुरे, तत्रबाधिर्यं।

(सु०शा०, 6/27)

Karnaprishthatoadhah sanshrite vidhure, tatrabadhiryam

(Su. Sharir, 6/27)

This marm lies on the lower side of the root of the ear (on the posterior and inferior border of the Mastoid process on the posterior border of sternocliedomastoid).

1. Name of the Marm	Vidhur Marm
2. Type of Marm	Snayu Marm
3. Prognosis	Vaikalyakar*
4. Quality Somya/Agneya	Somya
5. Size	Half angul (1.0 cm -1.5 cm)
6. Location	Sirabindu Shleshmashay 16, 17 (Sj 16, 17)
7. Indications	Deafness, Tinnitus *Tatra badhiryam*

According to *Sushrut Nidan*, 1/24, the causes of deafness are following:

श्रोत्रादिष्विन्द्रियवधं कुर्यात् क्रुद्धः समीरणः।

(सु०नि०, 1/24)

Shrotradishvindriyvadham kuryat kruddhah sameeranah

(Su. Nidan, 1/24)

Vitiated Vayu reaching the internal sense organs destroys its function leading to deafness.

Again Sushrut says in *Sushrut Nidan*, 1/83:

When vitiated vayu alone or mixed with Kaph surrounds the Auditory centres and gets fixed, causes immediate deafness. Damage of vestibulo cochlear nerve causes deafness or ringing in the ears.

यदा शब्दवहं स्रोतो वायुरावृत्य तिष्ठति।
शुद्धः श्लेष्मान्वितो वाऽपि बाधिर्यं तेन जायते।।

(सु०नि०, 1/83)

Yada Shabdavaham Sroto Vayuravrtya tisthati
Shuddhah shlesmanvito vapi badhiryam ten Jayate

(Su. Nidan, 1/83)

VIDHUR MARM, KAPHAJ DHAMANI AND SIRA OF URDHVAJATRU (SJ)
Sj: Sanjiao Channel (Yang)

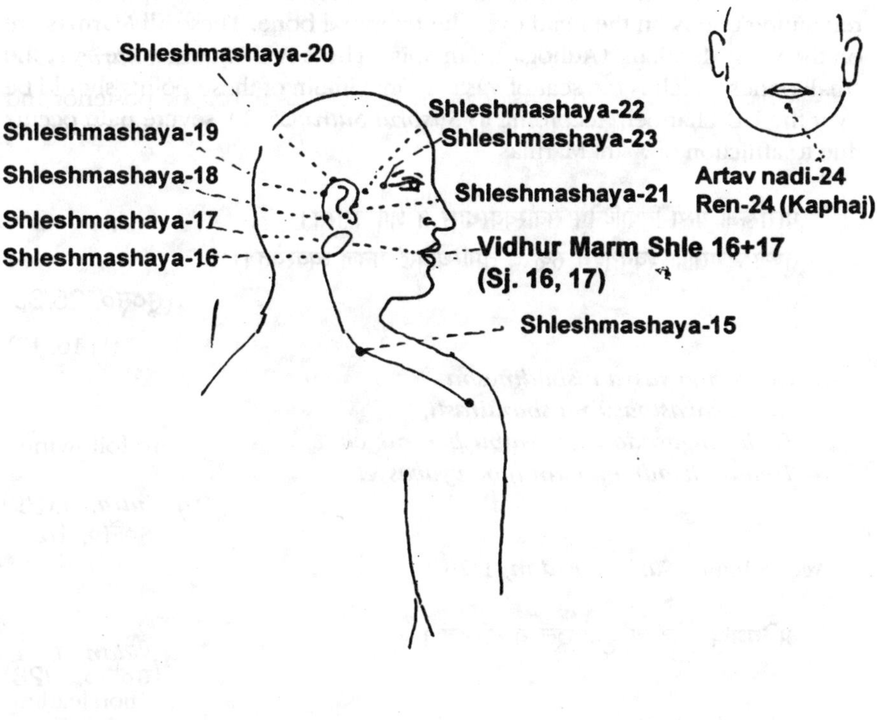

Figure 55

Asthi Marm

Asthi Marm are eight in number and are of four types.

Katiktarun	-	Two
Nitamb	-	Two
Ansaphalak	-	Two
Shankh	-	Two

Out of these four types of Asthi marmas, three are in back (pristh marm) remaining one is on the head over the temporal bone. These all Marmas are on the yang Meridians (Adhoga Dhamanis). These Asthi Marmas are over the small bones which is the seat of vasa. So maximum of these points should be over the UB Channel. According to *Sushrut Sutra,* 25/39, severe pain occurs due to affliction of Asthi Marmas.

घोरारूजो यस्य निषादिनेषु सर्वास्ववस्थासु न शान्तिरस्ति।
तृष्णाऽङ्गसादौ श्वयथुश्च रुक् च तमस्थिविद्धं मनुजं व्यवस्येत्।।

(सु०सू०, 25/39)

Ghorarujo yasya nishadineshu
Sarvasvavasthasu na shantirasti,
Trishnangasadou shvayathushch ruk ch
Tamasthividdham manujam vyavasyet.

(Su. Sutra, 25/39)

According to *Sushrut Nidan,* 1/28:

अस्थिशोषं प्रभेदं च कुर्याच्छूलं च तच्छितः।

(सु०नि०, 1/28)

Asthishosham prabhedam ch kuryat shulam ch tacchitah
(Su. Nidan, 1/28)

When the bone tissue is afflicted by vayu then it causes deterioration of function of bone marrow formation, etc. Shooting and piercing pain in the bone.

Katiktarun (Figure 56)

This Marm is the Marm of back (pristha marm) and is of Asthi Marm variety. According to *Su.Sh.*, 6/26

तत्र पृष्ठवंशमुभयतः प्रतिश्रोणिकाण्डमस्थिनी कटीकतरूणे
तत्र शोणितक्षयात् पाण्डुर्विवर्णो हीनरूपश्च म्रियते।

(सु०शा०, 6/26)

Tatra prishthvanshmubhayatah pratishronikandamasthini katiktarune
Tatra shonitkshayat pandurvivarno heenrupashch mriyate

(Su. Sharir, 6/26)

1. Name of the Marm	Katiktarun
2. Type of Marm	Asthi Marm.
3. Prognosis	Kalantar pranhar (death after sometime due to pain and loss of blood)
4. Quality Somya/Agneya	Somya + Agneya
5. Size	Half angul (1.0 cm –1.5 cm)
6. Location	First post sacral foramina Sira Mutrashay 31 + Mutrashay 53 (UB 31+UB53) (both sides)
7. Indications :	Severe pain over lumber region (low back pain) Haemorrhoids Uterine bleeding and pain, prolapse uterus.

For the above mentioned diseases, Siravedhan (acupuncture) of UB31+UB53 Sira is recommended.

MARM AND VATAJ, PITTAJ, KAPHAJ AND RAKTAJ SIRAS OF PRISHTHA (BACK)

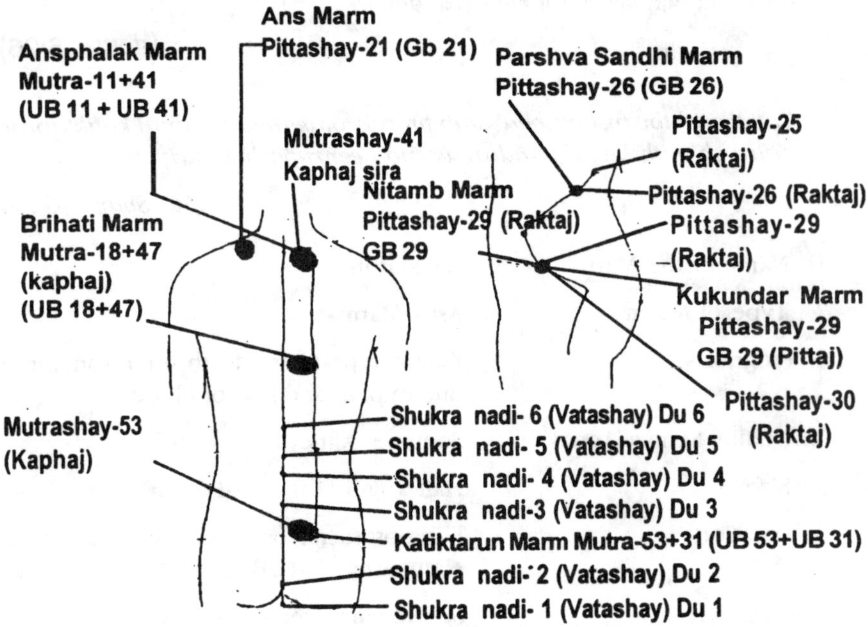

Figure 56

Nitamba Marm (Figure 57)

This is Marm of back (Pristhamarm) and is of Asthimarm variety. According to *Su.Sh.*, 6/26:

श्रोणिकाण्डयोरुपर्याशयाच्छादनौ पार्श्वान्तर प्रतिबद्धौनितम्बौ,
तत्राधःकायशोषो दौर्बल्याच्च मरणं।

(सु०शा०, 6/26)

Shronikandayoruparyashayachchadanou parshvantar pratibaddhou Nitambou, tatradhahkayashosho dourbalyachch maranam

(Su. Sharir, 6/26)

When this marm is damaged, there is atrophy of muscles of the lower extremities leading to impairment of functions of the lower part of body with general debility.

1. Name of the Marm	Nitamb Marm
2. Type of Marm	Asthi Marm
3. Prognosis	Kalantar Pranhar
4. Quality Somya/Agneya	Somya + Agneya
5. Size	Half angul (1.0 cm –1.5 cm)
6 Location	Sirabindu Pittashay 29 (GB29)
7. Indications	Paralysis of the lower extremities. Pain in the back and lower extremities.

The Nitamb Marm lies above and anterior to the sacrum, covering uterus and attached at the sides. When this Marm is damaged, there is atrophy of the muscles of lower extremities leading to impairment of function of the lower part of body with general debility.

Pittashay 29 (GB29) is Pittaj as well as Raktaj Sira therefore for Nitamb Marm it is used as Raktaj Sira while for Kukundar Marm it is used as Pittaj Sira.

MARM AND VATAJ, PITTAJ, KAPHAJ AND RAKTAJ SIRAS OF PRISHTHA (BACK)

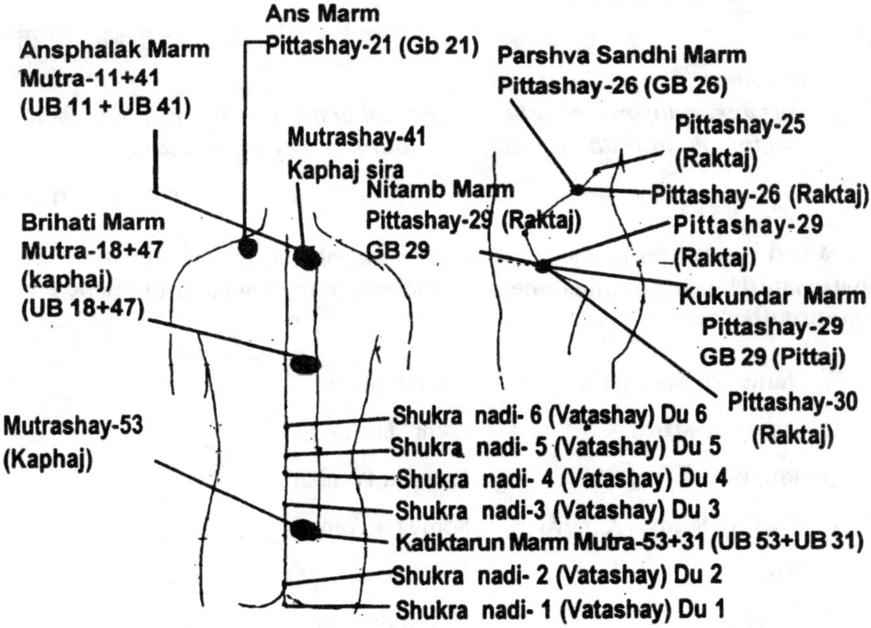

Figure 57

Ansphalak Marm (Figure 58)

This is also Asthi Marm. According to *Su.Sb.*, 6/26:

पृष्ठोपरि पृष्ठवंशमुभयतस्त्रिकसंबद्धे अंसफलके,
तत्र बाह्वोः स्वापशोषौ।

(सु०शा०, 6/26)

Prishthopari pristhvanshamubhayatastriksambaddhe ansphalake,
Tatra bahvoh svapshoshou

(Su. Sharir, 6/26)

Ansphalak Marm lies on the upper back of the vertebral column on both sides and is related to upper and middle part of scapula (TRIK) When this marm is afflicted, the muscles of the upper extremities get atrophied and the extremity becomes numb.

1. Name of the Marm	Ansphalak Marm
2. Type of Marm	Asthi Marm
3. Prognosis	Kalantar Pranhar
4. Quality Somya/Agneya	Somya + Agneya
5. Size	Half angul (1.0 cm –1.5 cm)
6. Location	Sirabindu Mutrashay11 + Mutrashay41 (UB11 +UB41) 1.25 inches lateral to the lower border of the Spinous process of the first thoracic vertebra. UB41-just below and lateral to it.
7. Indications	Arthritis and numbness of the upper Limbs. Tuberculosis of the bone. Brachial Neuritis.

The Sirabindu of this Marm is definitely UB11 due to its brachial plexus involvement. The word "Trik Sambaddhe" and its indication in the above shloka indicates its position in upper 1/3 of trik formed by both sides of upper part of Scapular blades and the first thoracic vertebra.

Both Siravedhan (Acupuncture) and Agnikarm (Moxibustion) are recommended.

MARM AND VATAJ, PITTAJ, KAPHAJ AND RAKTAJ SIRAS OF PRISHTHA (BACK)

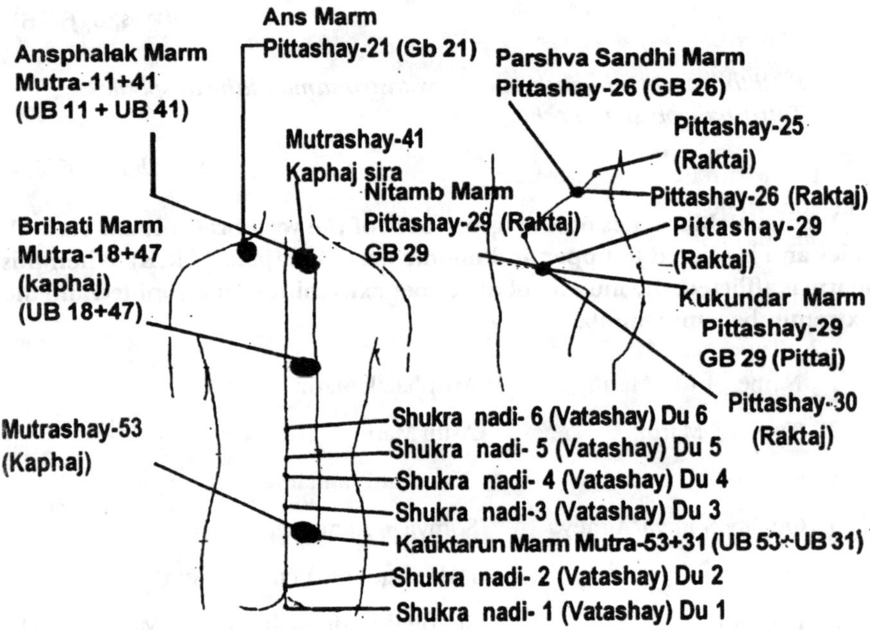

Figure 58

Shankh Marm (Figure 59)

This is the Urdhvajatru Marm (above clavicle) and is also Asthi Marm. According to *Su.Sh*, 6/27:

भ्रुवोरन्तयोरुपरि कर्णललाटयोर्मध्ये शङ्खौ, तत्रसद्योमरणं।

(सु०शा०, 6/27)

Bhruvorantayorupari karnlalatayormadhye shankhou, tatrasadyomaranam.

(Su. Sh., 6/27)

This Marm lies on upper part of the end of eyebrow and the centre of the line drawn on the upper part of the ear lobule to the forehead. The involvement of this Marm leads to sudden death.

1. Name of the Marm	Shankh Marm
2. Type of Marm	Asthi Marm
3. Prognosis	Sadya Pranhar (sudden death)
4. Quality Somya /Agneya	Agneya
5. Size	*Svapanital* 2 inches in diameter
6. Location	This is an extra point. (Location given above)
7. Indications	As below.

This marm is not on regular channel but it belongs to extra channel. According to *Sushrut Sharir*, 6/27, Utkshep is above this Marm. It is an area between Utkshep on the upper part and Apang Marm below. This area (temporal) is highly innervated by the sensory root of the Trigeminal nerve causing shock and death due to severe pain. Besides underneath this thin temporal bone is the temporal artery and its injury causes brain haemorrhage leading to instant death (Sadya pranhar). This is a famous point of Criminal *Hathori mar. This Marm has been missed in the original translation of *Sushrut Sanhita* by Chinese.

Note:

*Hathori mar was a self-styled criminal of India who hit a person fatally on temporal aspect of the head with hammer.

MARM, PITTAVAHINI DHAMANI AND SIRA OF URDHVAJATRU (ABOVE CLAVICLE)

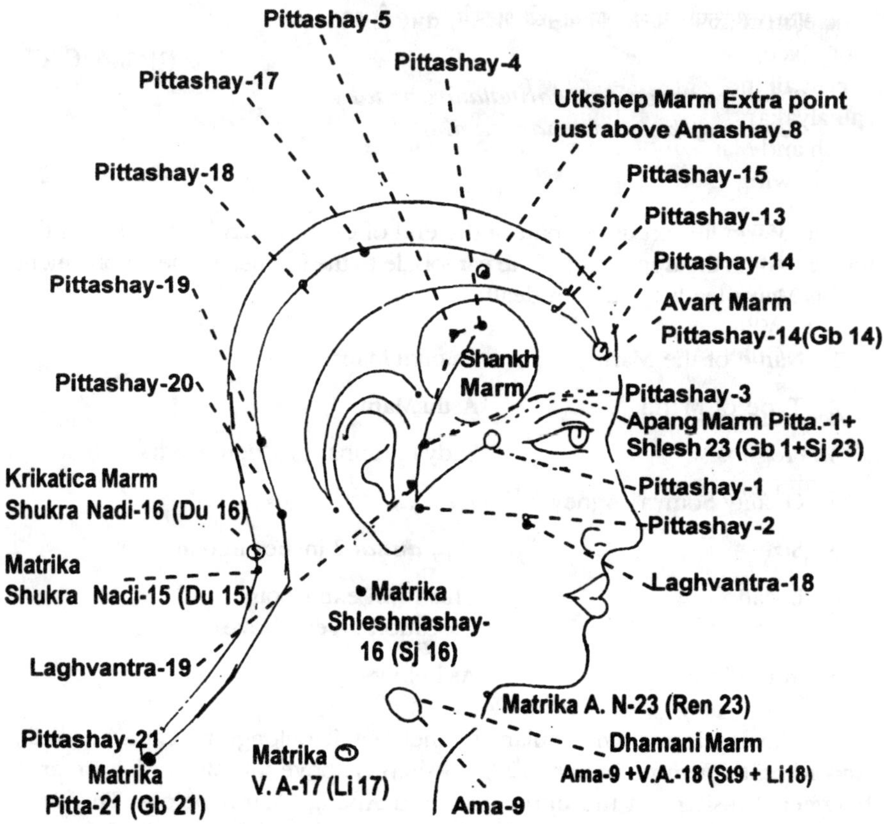

Figure 59

Sandhi Marm

All the Sandhi Marms are situated in joints, therefore they are called Sandhi Marmas.

According to *Su. Sutra,* 25/38, when the Sandhi Marmas are afflicted there is increase of inflammation and intense pain and loss of function of the effected joint. Except Adhipati Marm none of the Sandhi Marmas are Sadya pranhar. Almost all these Marmas come in the group of Kalantar pranhar, Rujakar and Vaikalyakar. Many of them are Somya and some are Somya+Agneya. Only Gulph and Manibandh are of Agni+Vayu Quality.

Following are the Sandhi Marmas:

Janu	Manibandh
Kurpar	Kukundar
Simant	Avart
Adhipati	Krikatia
Gulph	

According to *Sushrut Nidan,* 1/28:

हन्ति संधिगतः सन्धीन् शूलशोफौ करोति च ।

(सु०नि०, 1/28)

Hanti sandhigatah sandheen shoolshofou karoti ch.

(Su. Nidan, 1/28)

Janu Marm (Figure 60)

According to *Su.Sh.*, 6/24

जङ्घोर्वोः सन्धाने जानु, तत्र खञ्जता ।

Janghorvoh sandhane janu, tatra khanjata.

The Janu Marm lies between Leg and thigh. Its involvement causes lameness.

1. Name of the Marm	Janu Marm
2. Type of Marm	Sandhi Marm
3. Prognosis	Vaikalyakar
4. Quality Somya/Agneya	Somya + Agneya
5. Size	Three Angul (6.0 cm --9.0 cm)
6. Location	Sirabindu Pittashay 34, Mutrashay 40, Amashay 35 (GB34, UB40, St35).
7. Indications	Hemeplegia, Motor impairment of lower extremity.

MARM AND ADHOGA AMASHAY DHAMANI
Purush Sangyak (Yang)
St : Stomach Channel (Yang)

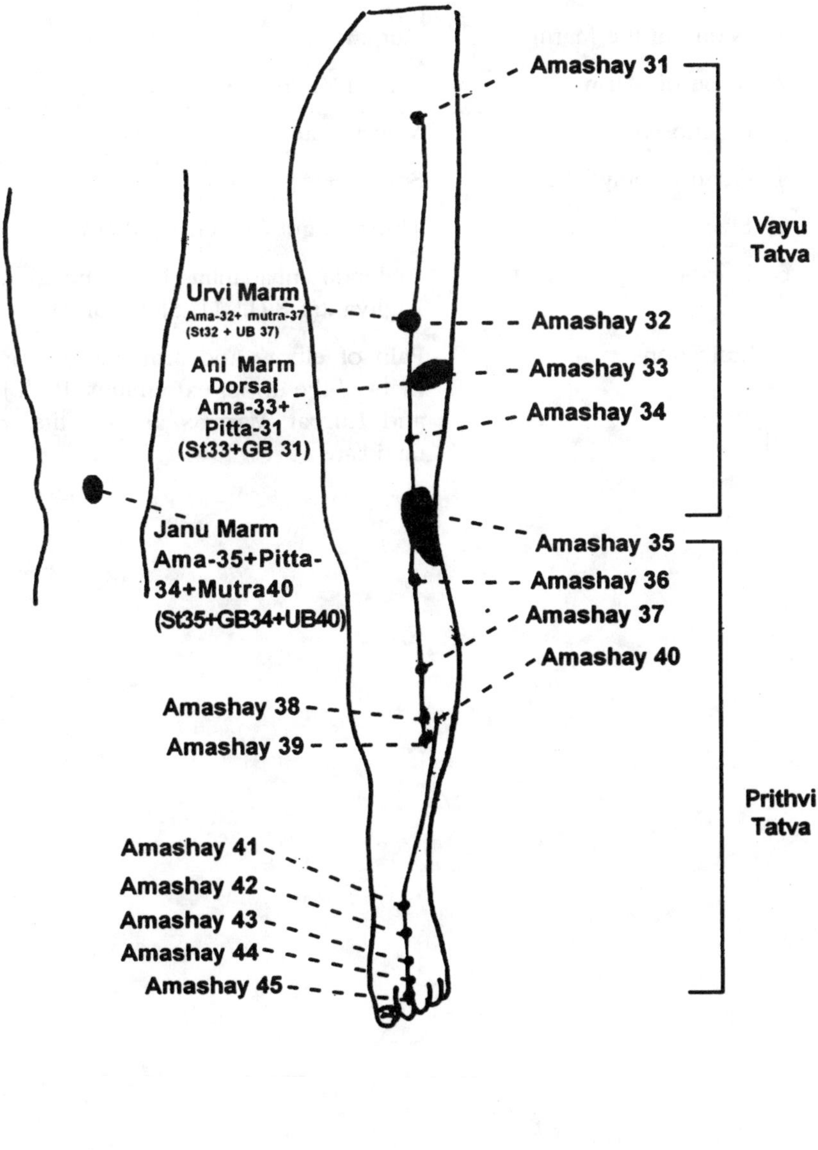

Figure 60

Kurpar Marm (Figure 61)

Kurpar is the Marm of upper extremity same as Janu Marm in the lower extremity, therefore the damage to this Marm causes pain of elbow and arm and motor impairment.

1. Name of the Marm	Kurpar
2. Type of Marm	Sandhi Marm
3. Prognosis	Vaikalyakar
4. Quality Somya/Agneya	Somya + Agneya
5. Size	Three Angul (6.0 cm –9.0 cm)
6. Location	Sirabindu Vrihadantra 11, Shleshmashay 10, Laghvantra 8 (LI 11, SJ 10, SI 8)
7. Indications	Pain of elbow and arm, motor impairment of the upper extremities. Both Janu and Kurpar Marmas are on the yang meridians.

ADHOGA LAGHVANTRA DHAMANI (RAKTASHAY AND PITTASHAY) PURUSH SANGYAK, KURPAR AND MANIBANDH MARM

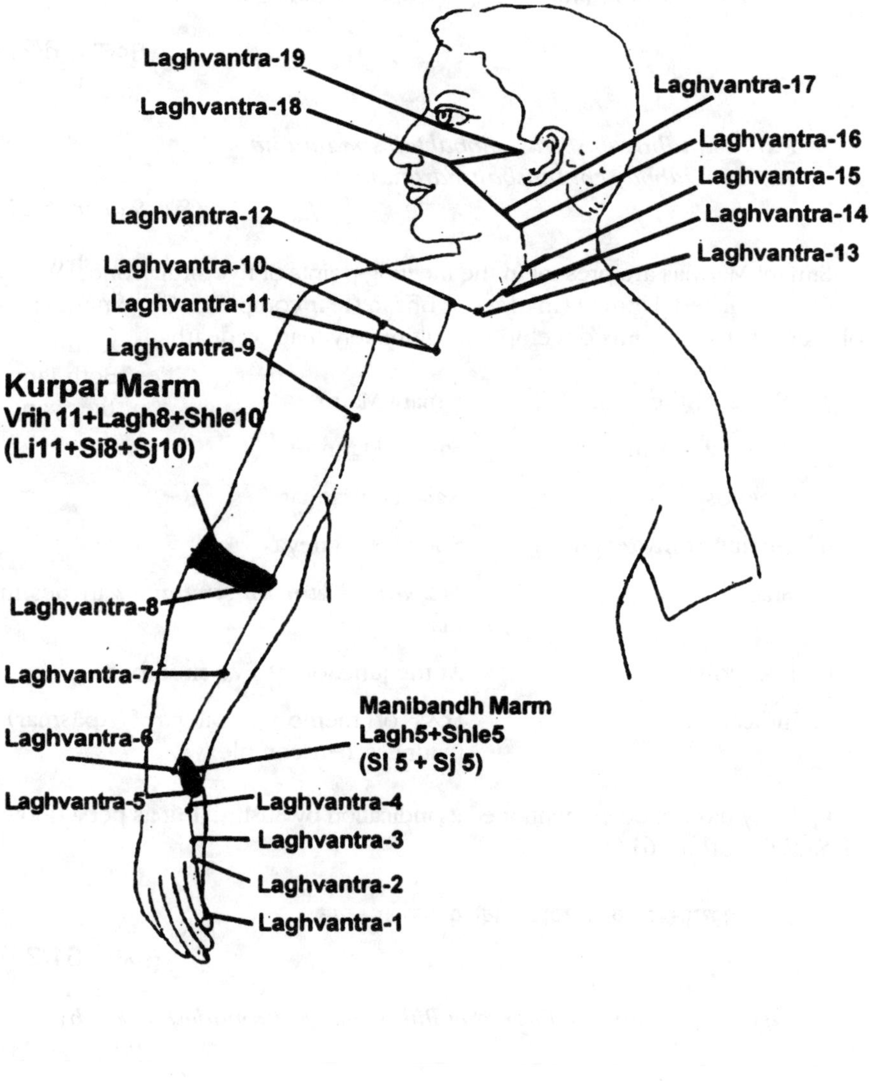

Figure 61

Simant Marm (Figure 62)

This is the Marm of Urdhvajatru (Head) and are of Sandhi Marm variety. According to *Su. Sharir*, 6/27

पञ्चसन्धयः शिरसि विभक्ताः सीमन्ता नाम, तत्रोन्मादभय चित्तनाशैर्मरणं।

(सु०शा०, 6/27)

Panchsandhayah shirasi vibhaktah simanta nam,
Tatronmadbhay chittnashairmaranam.

(Su. Sharir, 6/27)

Simant Marmas are present in the meeting points of five skull bones. When they are afflicted, Unmad (madness), Bhaya (fear complex), Chittanash (loss of memory) symptoms develop and ultimately lead to death.

1. Name of the Marm — Simant Marm
2. Type of Marm — Sandhi Marm
3. Prognosis — Kalantar pranhar
4. Quality Somya/Agneya — Somya + Agneya
5. Size — *Svapanital kunchit sammit* (2 inches in diameter)
6. Location — At the junction of five skull bones.
7. Indications — Loss of memory, epilepsy (Apasmar), madness, fear complex

Epilepsy has not been mentioned as indication by Sushrut but as per a quote of *Sushrut Uttar.*, 61/23

तस्य (अपस्मारस्य) कार्यो विधिः सर्वो य उन्मादेषुवक्ष्यते

(सु०उ०, 61/23)

Tasya (Apasmarasya) karyo vidhih sarvo ya unmadeshu vakshyate

(Su. Uttar., 61/23)

Stimulation of this Marm is done at the vertex one finger posterior, anterior and lateral, respectively at Shukra nadi 20 (DU20) point but according to Sushrut the method of stimulation should be by Agnikarm (Moxibustion) (permanent scarification) and not by siravedhan (Acupuncture).

तत्रशिरोरोगाधिमन्थयोर्भ्रूललाटशंङ्खप्रदेशेषु दहेत् ।

(सु०सू०, 12/9)

Tatra shirorogadhimanthayorbhru lalat shankh pradesheshu dahet

(Su. Sutra, 12/9)

Apply moxibustion in specific point of eyebrow, forehead and temporal area for the specific diseases of brain and eyes.

This Marm lies at the junction of five bones so by heat stimulation the brain is directly stimulated which is akin to modern Electric shock for various mental disorders. Accordingly it seems the method of Sushrut for madness is far superior than the modern method which is painful and dangerous as well. Besides above indications this Marm is also utilized by Sushrut in the treatment of snake bite.

......तीक्ष्णशस्त्रेण मूर्ध्नि च कृत्वा काकपदं चर्म सासृग्वा पिशितं क्षिपेत् ।......

(सु०कल्प, 5/23)

........Tikshnashastren murdhni ch kritva kakpadam
charm sasrigva pishitam kshipet.........

(Su. Kalp, 5/23)

In case of snake bite make a claw of crow like structure on the vertex by a sharp instrument and then apply fresh flesh on it. [This shows the use of Seemant Marm (which have five points seems like claw) in snake bite, epilepsy and unconciousness].

This point is not on the regular channel and is point of extra channel.

SIMANT AND ADHIPATI MARM

"Panch Sandhayah Shirasi Vibhaktah Simanta nam, Tatronmad bhay chittan-asheirmaranam" (*Sushrut Sharir*, 6/27)

"Mastakabhyantaroparishtat Sirasandhisannipato romavarto adhipatih" (*Sushrut Sharir*, 6/27)

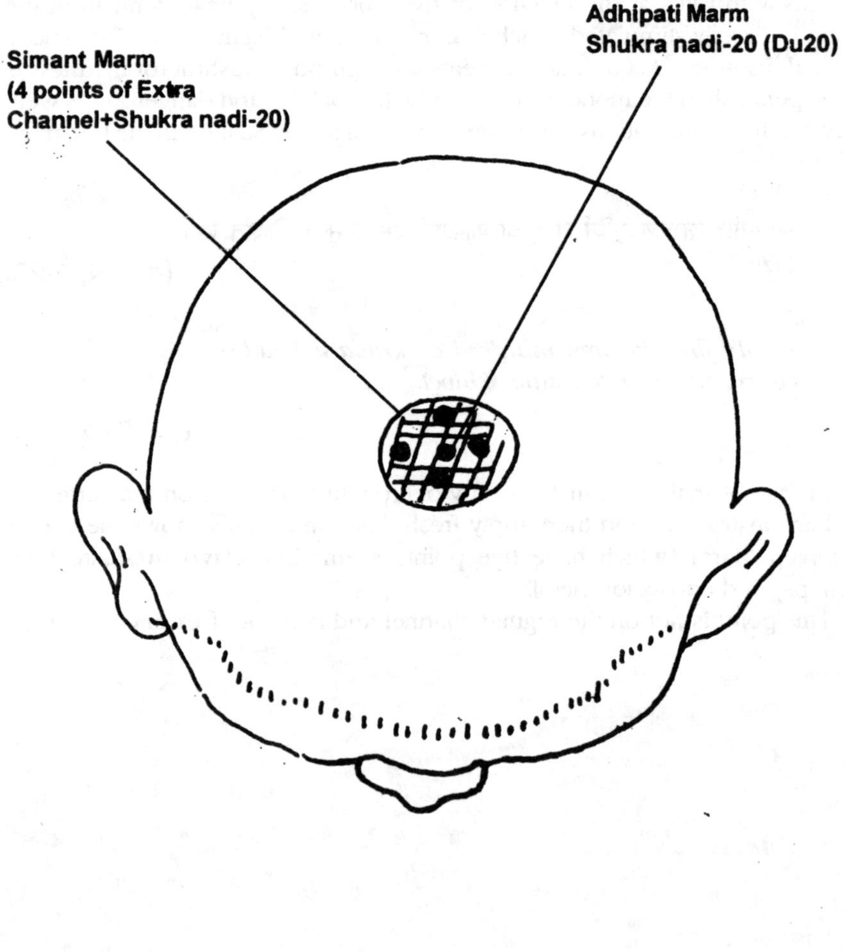

Figure 62

Adhipati Marm (Figure 63)

This is the Marm of Urdhvajatru over the centre of skull. According to *Su.Sb*, 6/27:

मस्तकाभ्यन्तरोपरिष्टात् सिरासन्धिसन्निपातो रोमावर्तोऽधिपतिः।

(सु०शा०, 6/27)

Mastakabhyantaroparishtat sirasandhisannipato romavartoadhipatih.

(Su. Sharir, 6/27)

This Marm lies on the top of the centre of the vertex at the junction of the Siras and joints of the skull bones, at the centre of whirl of hair.

1. Name of the Marm		Adhipati
2. Type of Marm		Sandhi Marm
3. Prognosis		Sadya pranhar (Instant death)
4. Quality Somya/Agneya		Agneya
5. Size		Half angul (1.0 cm –1.5 cm)
6. Location		Sirabindu Shukra nadi 20 (Du20) on the midpoint of the line connecting the apexes of the two auricles.
7. Indications	:	Cerebrovascular accidents, Apoplexy.

This Marm lies at the centre of four Simant Marm, Sushrut refers Avart for Simant Marm and Du 20 (Adhipati) is in the centre of these four Simant Marmas.

This Marm is the governing centre of all channels, therefore it is known as Adhipati. It can be used with Simant Marm in schizophrenia, parkinsonism epilepsy and other mental disorders for better results. Chinese have described it also as Baihui which means meeting point of several points.

Method of stimulation: Agnikarm (Moxibustion)

According to *Su.Sutra*, 12/9:

तत्र शिरोरोगाधिमन्थयोर्भ्रूललाट शंङ्खप्रदेशेषु दहेत्।

(सु०सू०, 12/9)

Tatra shirorogadhimanthayorbhru lalat shankhpradesheshu dahet.

(Su. Sutra, 12/9)

Sushrut says for the application of Moxibustion in specific point of eyebrow, forehead and temporal area for the specific diseases of brain and eyes.

So according to Sushrut Agnikarm (Moxibustion) is the best method for stimulation of Adhipati Marm.

ADHIPATI AND SIMANT MARM

"Panch Sandhayah Shirasi Vibhaktah Simanta nam, Tatronmad bhay chittan-asheirmaranam" (*Sushrut Sharir*, 6/27)

"Mastakabhyantaroparishtat Sirasandhisannipato romavarto adhipatih" (*Sushrut Sharir*, 6/27)

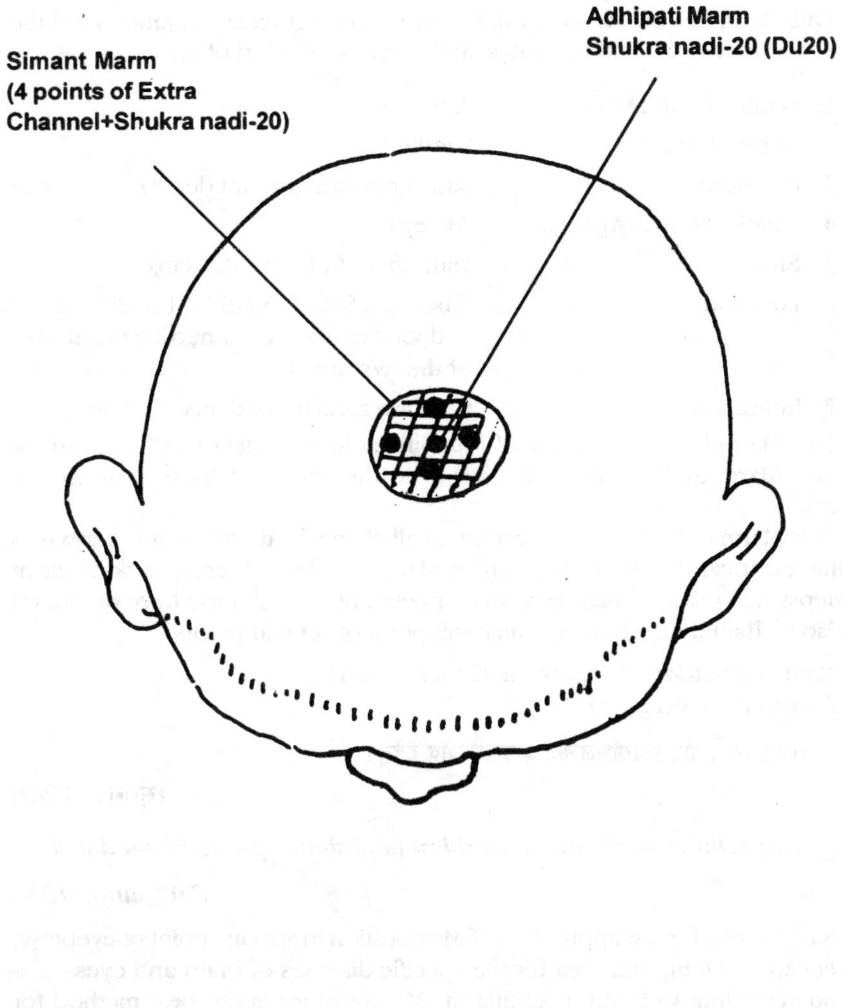

Figure 63

Gulph Marm (Figure 64)

This is the Marm of lower extremity located in the ankle joint. It is of Sandhi Marm variety, According to *Su. Sharir,* 6/24

पादजङ्घयोः सन्धाने गुल्फः तत्र रुजः स्तब्धपादता खञ्जता वा।

(सु०शा०, 6/24)

Padjanghyoh sandhane gulphah tatra rujah
stabdhapadata khanjata va.

(Su. Sharir, 6/24)

The Gulph Marm lies at the junction of foot with the leg. It is indicated for pain, numbness and limping.

1. Name of the Marm	Gulph Marm
2. Type of Marm	Sandhi Marm
3. Prognosis	Rujakar
4. Quality Somya/Agneya	Agni+Vayu ·
5. Size	Two Angul (4.0 cm –6.0 cm)
6. Location	Its point of cure Pittashay 39, Mutrashay 59 (GB39, UB59).
7. Indications	Weakness and paralysis of foot, hemiplegia, pain in the leg.

Method of stimulation:
Siravedhan (Acupuncture) half inch depth and Agnikarm (Moxibustion).

KURCH MARM, GULPH MARM AND PITTASHAY DHAMANI OF SAKTHI, PURUSH SANGYAK AND Gb: Gall-bladder Channel (Yang)

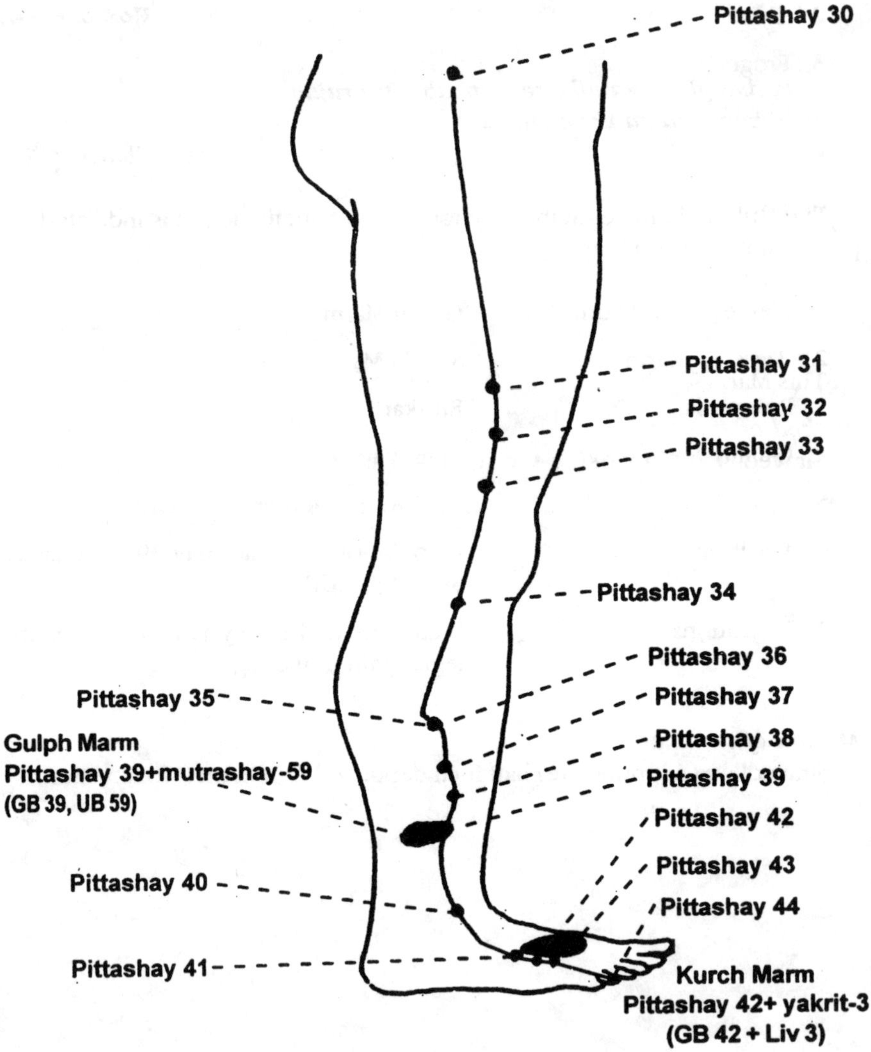

Figure 64

Manibandh Marm (Figure 65)

This is the Marm of upper extremity. Its location is on the wrist at the junction of hand with forearm.

1. Name of the Marm	Manibandh Marm
2. Type of Marm	Sandhi Marm
3. Prognosis	Rujakar
4. Quality Somya/Agneya	Agni+Vayu
5. Size	Two angul (4.0 cm –6.0 cm)
6. Location	Sirabindu Laghvantra 5, Shleshmashay 5 (SI 5, Sj 5).
7. Indications	Loss of function of wrist joint *Manibandhe kunthata* (*S.Sh.* 6/24)

This Marm is indicated in contraction and pain of elbow and arm.

Method of stimulation:
Siravedhan (Acupuncture) and Agnikarm (Moxibustion).

ADHOGA LAGHVANTRA DHAMANI (RAKTASHAY AND PITTASHAY) PURUSH SANGYAK, KURPAR AND MANIBANDH MARM

SI: Small Intestine Channel (Yang)

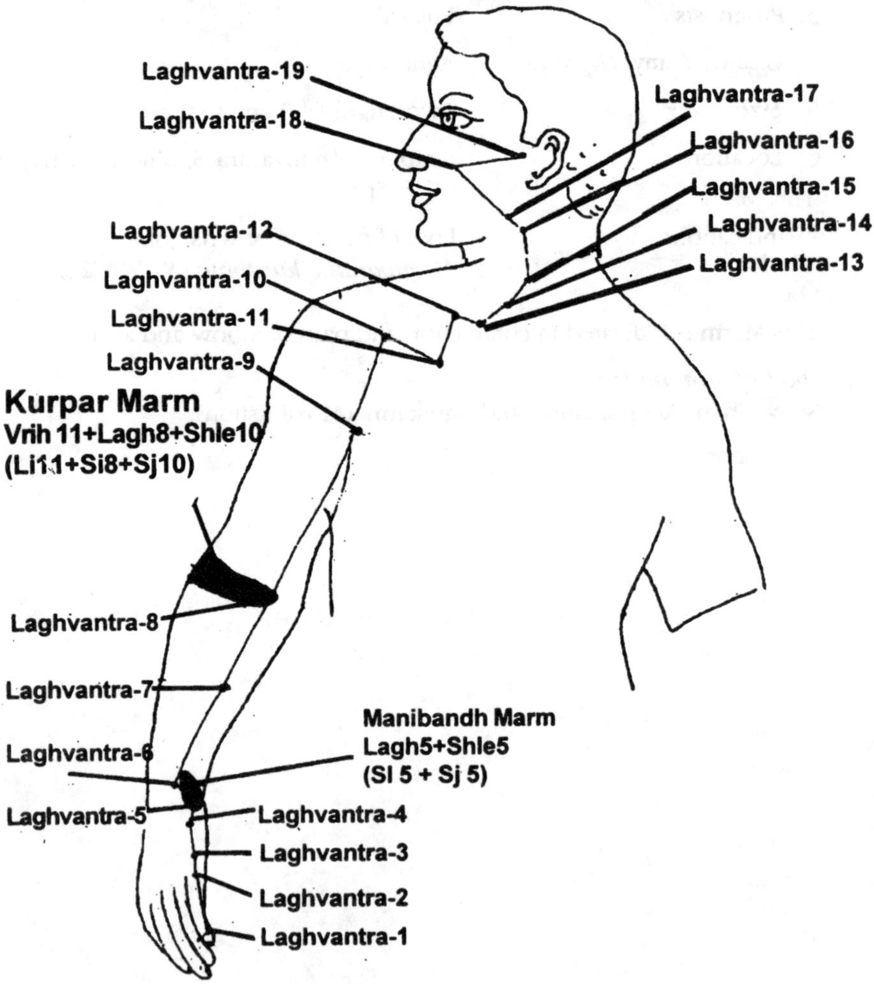

Figure 65

Kukundar Marm (Figure 66)

This Marm is of back and is of Sandhi marm variety. According to *Su. Sharir*, 6/26:

पार्श्वयोर्जघनबहिर्भागे पृष्ठवंशमुभयतो कुकुन्दरे,
तत्रस्पर्शाज्ञानमधःकाये चेष्टोपघातश्च।

(सु०शा०, 6/26)

Parshvayorjaghanbahirbhage prishthvanshamubhayato kukundare,
Tatrasparshagyanamadhahkaye cheshtopghatashch.

(Su.Sharir, 6/26)

This Marm lies on the lateral part of the hip joint on the outer side of the buttock, on the either side of the spinal cord. When this Marm is afflicted, it causes loss of sense of touch and impairment of function of the lower part of the body.

1. Name of the Marm	Kukundar Marm
2. Type of Marm	Sandhi Marm
3. Prognosis	Vaikalyakar (loss of function)
4. Quality Somya/Agneya	Somya + Agneya
5. Size	Half angul (1.0–1.5 cm)
6. Location	Pittashay29 (GB 29) of both sides.
7. Indications	Given below.

This Marm seems to be related with Sciatic nerve palsy which is different from Sciatic Neuritis or Sciatica. The Sciatic Nerve originates from the fourth and fifth lumbar and first and second Sacral roots. When there is complete Sciatic Nerve paralysis, the knee cannot be flexed and all muscles below the knee are paralysed. The nerve is commonly injured during fracture of pelvis or femur. The other causes are Pelvic-tumors, Diabetes Mellitus, Polyarteritis nodosa, Ruptured Lumbar Disc. Sensory loss is due to compression of Sciatic Nerve.

MARM AND VATAJ, PITTAJ, KAPHAJ AND RAKTAJ SIRAS OF PRISHTHA (BACK)

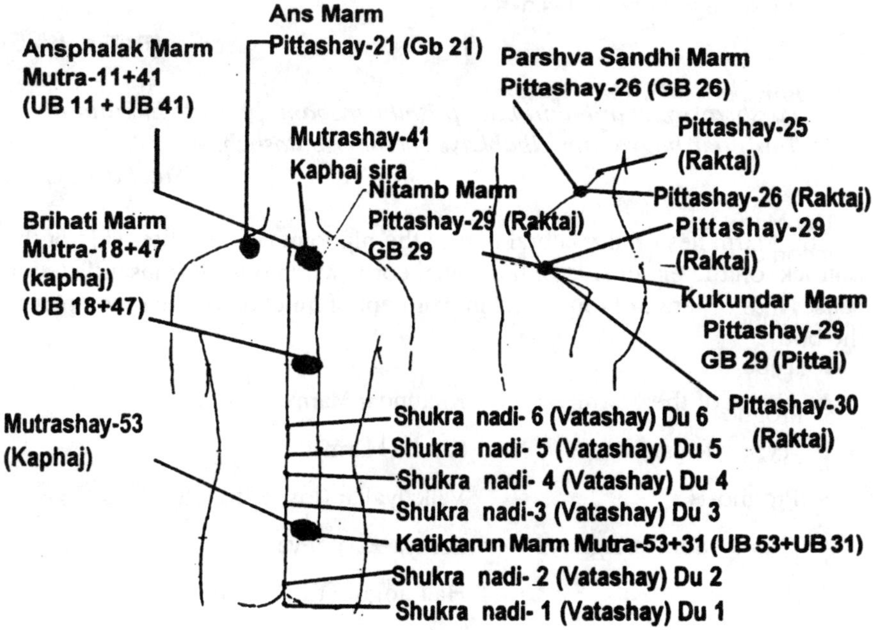

Figure 66

Avart Marm (Figure 67)

This is the Marm of Urdhvajatru present on the either side of the forehead. According to *Su.Sharir*, 6/27

भ्रुवोरुपरिनिम्नयोरावर्तो नाम तत्राप्यान्ध्यं दृष्ट्युपघातो वा।

(सु०शा०, 6/27)

Bhruvoruparinimnayoravarto nam
tatrapyandhyam drishtyupghato va.

(Su. Sharir, 6/27)

The Marm lies just above the eyebrows on the lower part of the forehead, affliction of which causes blindness and vision defects.

1. Name of the Marm	Avart Marm
2. Type of Marm	Sandhi Marm
3. Prognosis	Vaikalyakar (loss of function)
4. Quality Somya/Agneya	Somya + Agneya
5. Size	Half angul (1.0 cm –1.5 cm)
6. Location	Sirabindu Pittashay 14 (GB14) on the forehead 3/4th an inch above the mid-point of the eyebrow.
7. Indications	Blurring of vision (Drishti Upghata) Blindness (Andhyam) Lacrimation due to exposure to wind Pain in the outer canthus.

Method of stimulation :
By Agnikarm (Moxibustion)

MARM, PITTAVAHINI DHAMANI AND SIRA OF URDHVAJATRU (ABOVE CLAVICLE)

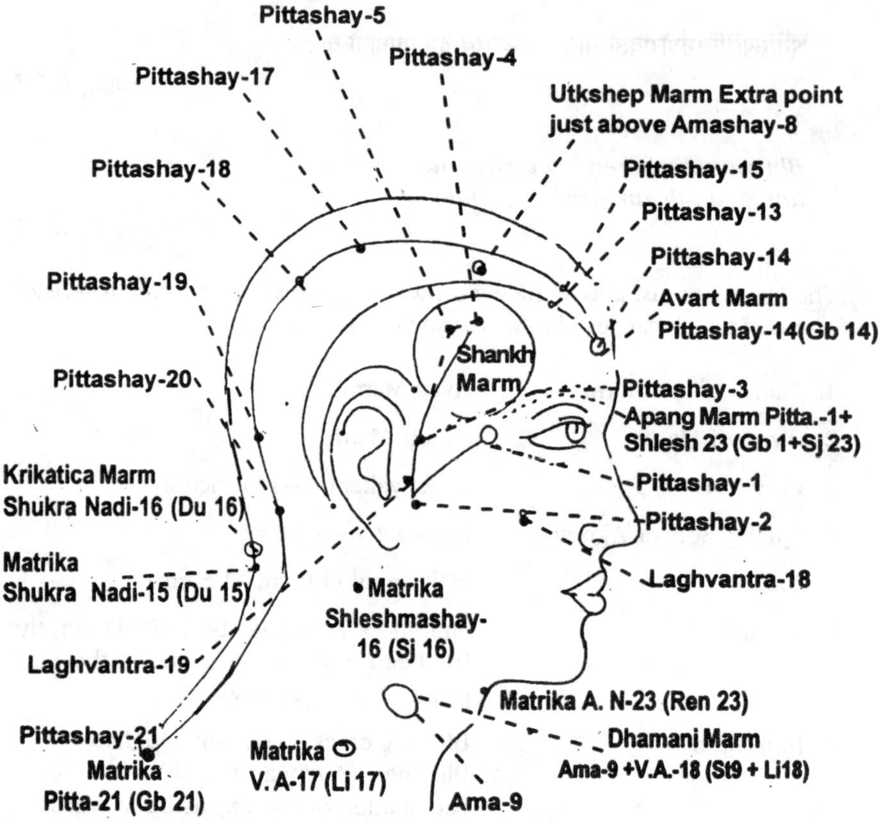

Figure 67

Krikatica Marm (Figure 68)

This is the Marm of Urdhvajatru (above the clavicle) on the back of the neck. According to *Su. Sharir*, 6/27:

शिरोग्रीवयोः सन्धाने कृकाटिके, तत्र चलमूर्धता।

(सु०शा०, 6/27)

Shirogreevayoh sandhane krikatike, tatra chalamurdhata

(Su. Sharir, 6/27)

This Marm lies at the junction of neck with head. Affliction of this marm causes mental disorders.

1. Name of the Marm	Krikatica
2. Type of Marm	Sandhi Marm
3. Prognosis	Vaikalyakar
4. Quality Somya/Agneya	Somya + Agneya
5. Size	Half angul (1.0 cm –1.5 cm)
6. Location	Sirabindu Shukranadi 15, 16 (DU 15, 16), DU 15 - In the midpoint of the Nape with in the hair line. DU16 - Directly below the external occipital protuberance.
7. Indication	Mental Disorders, Epilepsy.

Both of these Marmas are related to Avyavasthit Chitta (mental abberrations and mental disorders).

Sushrut has forbidden puncturing (Avedhya Sira), so Agnikarm (Moxibustion) is indicated.

MARM, PITTAVAHINI DHAMANI AND SIRA OF URDHVAJATRU (ABOVE CLAVICLE)

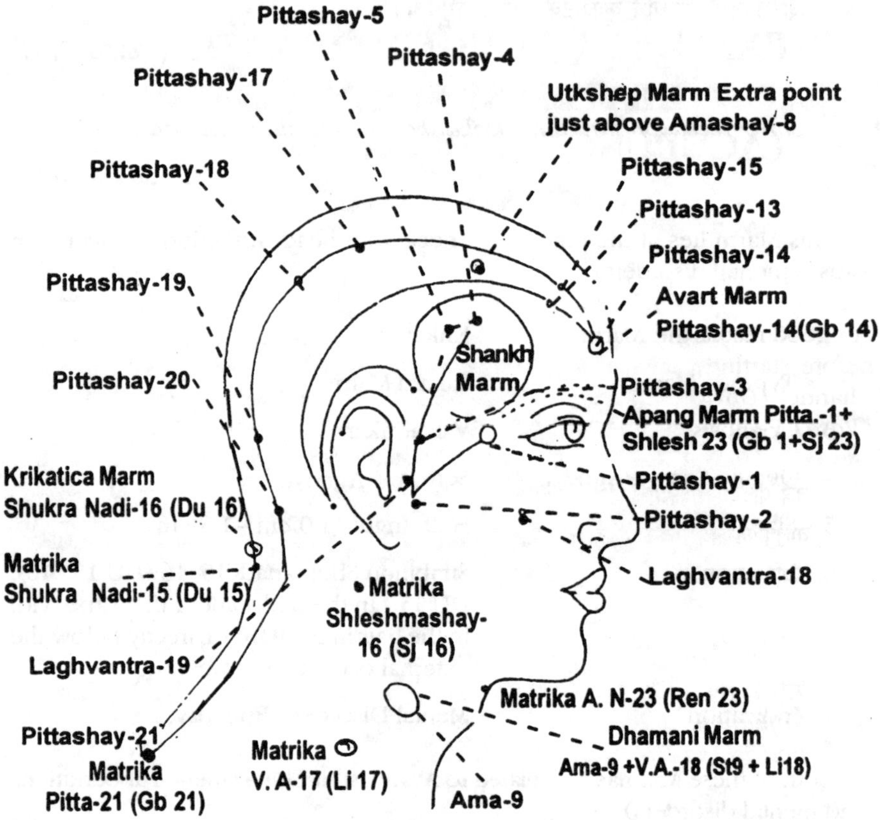

Figure 68

Chapter 8

EXAMPLES OF COMMON DISEASES TREATED BY SIRAVEDHAN (ACUPUNCTURE) AND AGNIKARM (MOXIBUSTION)

For good results Snehan (oleation) and Svedan (Sudation) must be performed before starting principal karm. Snehan and Svedan are performed by DU Channel *(Ghrit),* Ren channel *(Tail),* Kidney channel *(Majja),* UB Channel *(Vasa),* P-Channel (P4- *Agni (swedan))*

तत्र पाददाहपादहर्षचिप्पविसर्पवातशोणित
वातकण्टकविचर्चिकापाददारीप्रभृतिषु क्षिप्रमर्मण
उपरिष्टाद् व्यड.गुले व्रीहिमुखेन सिरां विध्येत्।

(सु०शा०, 8/17)

Tatra pad-dah pad-harsh chippa visarp vatshonit
Vatkantak vicharchika pad-dari prabhritishu kshipramarman
uparishtad Vyadyangule vreehimukhen siram vidhyet

(Su.Sharir, 8/17)

In the following diseases Acupuncture (Siravedhan) should be done on the recommended points, two fingers in breadth above the Kshipra Marm Talhridaya 8 (p8) and Vrikka 1, 2 (K1,2).

Pad-dah: In *Su. Nidan,* 1/80, it is defined as follows:

When the vitiated Vayu combines with Rakta and Pitta are vitiated causes burning sensation on the sole.

Pad-harsh: When Kapha and Vata both are vitiated it causes tingling and numbness in both the legs.

Chippa: When Pitta and Vayu take shelter under nail flesh causes pain burning and pus formation. This is also called Upnakh. (ingrowing toe nail due to fungal infection of the nail). See *Su. Nidan,* 13/21

Visarpa: When all the three doshas (Kapha, Vayu and Pitta) are vitiated and get shelter together in skin, muscles and blood, it spreads in all the directions, resulting in swelling which is not visible as raised produces symptoms according to the dosh involved. (When Pitta is involved, the symptoms appear as in Herpes, when Kaph is involved it causes lot of itching, pus formation is late. All these symptoms show viral origin.)

Vatshonit: Due to multiple pittavardhak causes the vitiated Rakta obstructs the path of speedy Vayu. Due to obstruction in its pathway the highly vitiated Vayu highly vitiates Rakta,characterised by severe pain and inflammation in lower limbs specially big toe *(See Su. Nidan,* 1/41-44). It can be simulated with Gout.

Vatkantak: When Vayu in Gulpha Sandhi is vitiated, while placing foot on an uneven ground pain occurs.

Vicharchika: When there are fissure and cracks on the skin of hands and feet due to dryness it results in pain, itching and dryness.

Pad-dari: Vata causes Paddari on the sole of habitual walkers where skin is dry. *(See Su.Nidan,* 13/29).

Shlipad: When the three vitiated doshas descend down into the groin, thigh, knee and leg and get fixed there, gradual swelling occurs after sometime and it is called Shlipad.

Treatment of Vataj Shlipad: In *Sh. Chikitsa,* 19/52-54, Sushrat clarifies:

स्नेहस्वेदोपपन्ने तु श्लीपदेऽनिलजे भिषक्।
कृत्वा गुल्फोपरि सिरां विध्येत्तु चतुरङ.गुले।।

(सु०चि०, 19/52–54)

Snehsvedoppanne tu shlipade anilaje bhishak,
Kritva gulphopari siram vidhyettu chaturangule

(Su. Chikitsa, 19/52-54)

In Vataj Shlipad, stimulate the point Phiha 6 (SP6) as well Pliha 9 (SP9) which are in the same channel, four angul above the Gulpha Marm after Snehan and Svedan. (Snehan: Stimulation of Du, Ren, K and UB Channel. Svedan : Stimulation of point of pericardium channel specially P4.)

According to Sushrut, in above Shlok, after this process give Basti (by puncturing Mutrashay 20, 21, 39.(UB20, 21, 39) and then advises to continue stimulation of Artav nadi 6, 9 (Ren 6, 9) to perform the effect of drinking Castor Oil with Urine. For diet he advises to take Rice cooked in milk, decoction of ginger. Habitually use trivrit such as mentioned in vatvyadhi. Best method of stimulation in the disease is Agnikarm (Moxibustion).

Pittajanya Shlipad: As mentioned in *Su. Chi.*, 19/55:

गुल्फस्याधः सिरां विध्येच्छलीपदे पित्तसंभवे।
फ्तिघ्नीं च क्रियां कुर्यात् पित्तार्बुदविसर्पवत्

(सु०चि०, 19/55)

Gulphasyadhah siram vidhyechchhlipade pittasambhave,
Pittaghnim ch kriyam kuryat pittarbud visarpavat.

(Su. Chi., 19/55)

In Pittaj Shlipad puncture the Yang Siras below the Gulph Marm i.e. Pittashay 39, 40 (GB39, 40) and apply those procedures which reduce pitta as in Pittaj Tumors and Herpes. GB39, 40 being the son point reduces the enhanced pitta and its location is four fingers above the tip of External Malleolus.

Kaphaj Shlipad: In *Su. Chi*, 19/56, Acharya identifies:

सिरां सुविदितां विध्येदङ्गुष्ठे श्लैष्मिके भिषक्।

(सु०चि०, 19/56)

Siram suviditam vidhyedangushthe shleishmike bhishak

(Su. Chi., 19/56)

In Shleshmik Shlipad puncture the famous sira of toe i.e., Vrikka 1 (K1) K1 being the reducing point has been taken here for Kaphaj Shlipad. For Medicinal Treatment see further *Su. Chikitsa,* 19/56-62.

Kroshtukshirsha: (See *Su. Sharir,* 8/17):

क्रोष्टुकशिरः खञ्जपङ्गुलवातवेदनासु जङ्घायां गुल्फस्योपरि चतुरङ्गुले (सिरा विध्येत्)

(सु०शा०, 8/17)

Kroshtukshirah khanj pangul vatvedanasu
Janghayam gulphasyopari chaturangule (Sira Vidhyet)

(Su. Sharir, 8/17)

In the above said diseases the siravedhan should be done four angul above the Gulph Marm in the leg.

When both vayu and shonit get vitiated and get fixed in knee they cause inflammation and extreme pain. The swollen knee appears like the head of jackal.

The points are Pliha 7 (Sp 7), Amashay 40 (St 40), Pittashay 35 (GB 35), Yakrit 5 (Liv 5).

In these points Sp7 and St40 are vayu points to reduce vayu and GB35 and LIV5 are shonit points to reduce the shonit.

Khanj and Pangul: As curative points are indicated in *Su. Nidan,* 1/77:

वायुः कट्यां स्थितः सक्थनः कण्डरामाक्षिपेद्यदा।
खञ्जस्तदा भवेज्जन्तुः पङ्गुः सक्थ्नोर्द्वयोर्वधात्।।

(सु० नि०, 1/77)

Vayuh katyam sthitah sakthnah kandaramakshipedyada
Khanjastada bhavejjantuh panguh sakthnordvayorvadhat.

(Sushrut Nidan, 1/77)

When the vayu which is lodged in the groins causes loss of function at the big ligament or big nerves (sciatic nerve) of lower extremity, it causes khanj (limping). When it effects both the Kandaras of lower extremities then patient becomes Pangu (motionless). The curative points are same as in Kroshtuk Shirsha.

Vatvedana: For curative points, see *Su. Sh.,* 8/17:

When vayu alone is involved it causes Vatvedana (Vatik pain). The curative points again are same as mentioned above ie Vataj points as Pliha 7 (Sp7) and Amashay 40 (St40).

Apachi: For location of points, see *Su. Sh.,* 8/57:

अपच्यामिन्द्रबस्तेरधस्ताद् व्यङ्गुले।

(सु० शा०, 8/17)

Apachyamindrabasteradhastad vdyangule

(Su. Sharir, 8/17)

In Apachi (cervical lymphadenitis, tubercular adenitis and scrofula) the siravedhan, scarification and Agnikarm points are two angul below the Indravasti Marm of both upper and lower extremities, i.e.

Pittashay 38 (GB 38) in lower extremities
Laghvantra 5 (SI 5) in upper extremities

Sh. Chi, 18/25-27 shows the same location of sirabindu for Apachi.

पार्ष्णि प्रति द्वे दश चाङ्गुलानि।
भित्वेन्द्रबस्ति परिवर्ज्य धीमान्।
मणिबन्धोपरिष्टाद्वा कुर्याद्रेखात्रयं भिषक्।
अंङ्गुल्यन्तरितं सम्यगपचीनां निवृत्तये

(सु०चि०, 18/25, 27)

Parshni prati dve dash changulani,
Bhitvendra basti parivarjya dheeman
Manibandhoparishtadva kuryadrekhatrayam bhishak
Angulyantaritam samyagapachinam nivrittaye

(Su. Chikitsa, 18/25,27)

Acharya recommends three lines of Scarification over the Manibandh area i.e. points on SI, SJ and LI channel (Laghvantra 5, Shleshmashay 6, Vrihadantra 6—SI 5, SJ 6, LI 6).

Gridhrasi: Acharya has said in *Su. Sharir,* 8/17:

जानुसंधेरुपर्यधो वा चतुरङ्गुले गृध्रस्यां।

(सु०शा०, 8/17)

Janusandheruparyadho va chaturangule gradhrasyam

(Su. Sharir, 8/17)

***Definition of Gridhrasi*:** According to *Su. Nidan,* 1/74:

पार्ष्णिप्रत्यङ्गुलीनां तु कण्डरा याऽनिलार्दिता।
सक्थ्नः क्षेपे निगृह्णीयाद् गृध्रसीति हि सा स्मृता।।

(सु०नि०, 1/74)

Parshnipratyangulinam tu kandara ya anilardita
Sakthnah kshepe nigraniyad gridhrasiti hi sa smrita

(Su. Nidan, 1/74)

It involves the big nerves over the dorsum of the foot, ankle joint and over every metatarsals causing pain and motionlessness of leg.

It shows involvement of the lower part of Sciatic Nerve.

Sciatic Nerve is derived from L4, L5 and S1, S2 roots. It provide the motor innervation of the hamstring muscles and all muscles below the knee.In

Gridhrasi the common peroneal branch of Sciatic nerve is involved:

Amashay 33 (ST 33)	-	Four angul above the laterosuperior border of patella for motor impairment and numbness of lower extremity.
Amashay 37, 38 (ST37, 38)	-	Motor impairment, muscular atrophy and paralysis of the leg.
Mutrashay 56 (UB56)	-	3 inches below popliteal crease.
Pittashay 34 (GB34)	-	In the depression anterior and inferior to the head of fibula.
Pittashay 32 (GB 32)	-	In the lateral aspect of the thigh.

It is to be noted that when the disease is in the lower part, the points of correction are above (distant points) and vice-versa in Gridhrasi and kroshthuk shirsha.

Galgand: In *Su. Sharir*, 8/17, Acharya says:

ऊरुमूलसंश्रितां गलगण्डे, एतेनेतरसक्थि बाहू च व्याख्यातौ।

(सु० शा०, 8/17)

Urumulsanshritam galgande, aetenetarsakthi bahu ch vyakhyatou

(Su. Sharir, 8/17)

The points of Galgand are situated in Urumul, but in this case the shlok further says that we can take upper extremity for stimulation as points of lower extremity therefore we are taking Vrihadantra 17, 18 (LI 17, 18) and Shleshmashay 13 (Sj 13) i.e. area of Bahumool which is equivalent to Urumool. (Similarly he advises to take Pliha 9 (Sp 9) in the knee (Janu marm) as Talhriday 3 (P3) in kurpar both have Similar action in Plihodar)

Plihodar: Again in *Su. Sharir*, 8/17, Acharya clears:

विशेषतस्तु वामबाहौ कूर्परसन्धेरभ्यन्तरतो बाहुमध्येप्लीह्नि
कनिष्ठिकानामिकयोर्मध्ये वा।

(सु०शा०, 8/17)

Visheshtastu vambahou kurparsandherabhyantarato bahumadhye plehni Kanishthika anamikayormadhye va.

(Su. Sharir, 8/17)

For splenomegali either puncture or apply Agnikarm (Moxa) the Sira which is over the centre of the elbow joint and on the ventral aspect i.e. Talhriday 3 (P3).

Acharya Sushrut further says that for the same disease the point of siravedhan is in the centre of Ring finger and little finger i.e. Shleshmashay 2, 3 (SJ2, 3).

Yakridalyudar

दक्षिणबाहौ यकृद्दाल्ये (कफोदरे च)

Dakshinbahou yakriddalye (Kaphodare ch)

For Hepatomegali and Liver diseases the point of siravedhan is Laghvantra 4 (SI4). Another point for Hepatomegali is Shleshmashay 10 (Sj 10).

Kasa-Shvasa: Acharya in *Su. Sharir,* 8/17, identifies the exact location of points:

एतामेव च कास श्वासयोरप्यादिशन्ति

(सु० शा०, 8/17)

Etamev ch kasa shvasayorapyadishanti

(Su. Sharir, 8/17)

Similarly for Kasa-Shvasa take points in the Dorsum of the arm i.e. Phuffus 7 (LU7) which is located above the Styloid process of radius.

Vishvachi: For selection of points, see in *Su. Sharir,* 8/17:

गृध्रस्यामिव विश्वाच्यां

(सु० शा०, 8/17)

Gridhrasyamiv vishvachyam

(Su. Sharir, 8/17)

In Vishvachi the method of selection of points are same as in Gridhrasi i.e. the point above and below Kurpar Sandhi (Elbow joint)

Definition of Vishvachi (See *Su. Nidan,* 1/75): Involvement of the nerves of lower part of brachial plexus supplying small muscles of hand and fingers of both sides ie ventral and dorsal are involved leading to restriction of the movement of the fore arm.

Ulcerative collitis with Tenesmus: According to *Su. Sharir,* 8/17:

श्रोणिं प्रति समन्ताद् व्यङ्गुले प्रवाहिकायां शूलिन्यां।

(सु०शा०, 8/17)

Shronim prati samantad vdyangule pravahikayam shulinyam

(Su. Sharir, 8/17)

In ulcerative collitis tenesmus, puncture the points two fingers apart around the waist.

Following are the curative points:

Artav nadi 6 (Ren6), Vrikka 16 (K16), Pliha 15 (Sp15), Yakrit 13 (Liv13), Amashay 25 (St25), Pittashay 25 (GB25), Mutrashay 22 (UB22), Shukra nadi 5 (Du 5).

Similarly on the other half will complete the belt *(Shroni samantad)*.

Parivartika, updansh, Shukrog and Shukrarog

परिवर्तिकोपदंशशूकदोषशुक्र व्यापत्सु मेढ्रमध्ये

(सु०शा०, 8/17)

Parivartikopadansh shookdosh shukra uyapatsu medhramadhye

(Su. Sharir, 8/17)

Parivartika (Paraphymosis)

Upadansh: Inflammatory and ulcerative disease of the prepuce of penis due to various causes (see *Su. Ni.*, 12/7). It is not syphlitic chancre.

Shukdosh: Inflammation caused by application of irritants.

Shukra Vyapad: Shukra Vyapad includes diseases and abnormalities of semen, its discharge such as seminal emissions, impotency (see Su. Sharir, 8/17).

............शुक्रव्यापत्सु मेढ्रमध्ये।

(सु० शा०, 8/17)

............*Shukra vyapatsu medhramadhye*

(Su. Sharir, 8/17)

For all the above said diseases, the points of stimulation are in the centre of the root of the penis i.e. Artav nadi 2, 3 (Ren 2, 3) and Vrikka 11, 12 (K 11, 12).

Method of stimulation:

Siravedh (Acupuncture - 0.3 -0.5 inch) and Agnikarm (Moxibustion).

Mutravriddhi: For details, see *Su. Nidan, 12/4:*

अधः प्रकुपितोऽन्यतमो हि दोषः फलकोशवाहिनीरभिप्रपद्य।
धमनीः फलकोषयोर्वृद्धिं जनयति, तां वृद्धिमित्याचक्षते॥

(सु०नि०, 12/4)

Adhah prakupito anyatamo hi doshah phalkoshvahinirabhiprapadya,
Dhamaneeh phalkoshayorvriddhim janayati, tam vriddhimityachakshate

(Su. Nidan, 12/4)

After an attack of mumps, typhoid or gonococcal infection when this infection (dosh) descends through Phalkosh vahini dhamani i.e. epididymis and reaches the testis causing acute inflammation of both testis and epididymis. When untreated Scrotum becomes full with oedematus fluid giving an appearance of Mashak. For further details see *Su. Nidan,* 12/6.

The points of cure, according to *Su. Sharir,* 8/17 are:

वृषणयोः पार्श्वे मूत्रवृद्धयां

(सु०शा०, 8/17)

Vrishanayoh parshve mootravriddhayam

(Su. Sharir, 8/17)

Vrikka 11, Yakrit 12, Pliha 11 (K11, LIV12, SP11)

Method of stimulation:
Siravedhan (acupuncture 0.3-0.5 inch) and Agnikarm (Moxibustion).

Dakodar: Portal vein and related lymphatic channels - ***Sneha vahini.***

Definition: According to *Sushrut Nidan,* 7/21-23, when the Ambuvahi srot gets obstructed it leads to accumulation of excessive fluid within the peritoneal cavity, giving symptoms of ascitis: it is called Dakodar.

The curative points are as maintioned in *Su. Sharir,* 8/17:

नाभेरधश्चतुरङ्गुले सेवन्या वामपार्श्वे दकोदरे

(सु०शा०, 8/17)

Nabheradhashchaturangule sevanya vamparshve dakodare

(Su. Sharir, 8/17)

Yakrit 13 (LIV13) - Which is front mu point of spleen and is located below and four finger lateral to umblicus and Mutrashay 20 (UB20) which is the Backshu point of Spleen completes the Dwimukhi Nadi Dakodar Yantra.

***Method of stimulation*:**
Siravedhan (acupuncture) - 0.5 - 1.0"
and Agnikarm(Moxibustion).

Antarvidradhi and Parshvashool:

Antarvidradhi as such could not be followed properly. The Parshvashool is pain in chest and hypochondriac region and sensation of fulness, Asthma, General Aches and weakness.

According to *Su. Sharir*, 8/17, the curative points are:

वामपार्श्वे कक्षास्तनयोरन्तरेऽन्तर्विद्रधौ पार्श्वशूले च।

(सु०शा०, 8/17)

Vamparshve kaksha stanayorantare antarvidradhou parshvashoole ch.

(Su. Sharir 8/17)

According to above mentioned shlok the curative points are following: Pliha 19, 20, 21 (SP19, 20, 21).

***Method of stimulation*:**
Siravedhan (Acupuncture 0.3 - 0.5 inch) and Agnikarm (Moxibustion).

Bahushosh and Avabahuk: Acharya in *Su. Nidan*, 2/82 explains:

अंसदेशस्थितो वायुः शोषयित्वांऽसबन्धनम्।
सिराश्चाकुञ्च्य तत्रस्थो जनयत्यवबाहुकम्

(सु०नि०, 2/82)

Ans deshasthito vayuh shoshayitvamansbandhanam,
Sirashchakunchya tatrastho janayatyavabahukam

(Su. Nidan, 2/82)

When the vayu which is located in shoulder and scapular region affects the connections of the shoulder and scapular joint causing emaciations and atrophy of the related muscles and constricts the ligaments and motor path ways of the region - it is called Avabahuk and Bahushosh.

The corrective points as mentioned in *Su. Sharir,* 8/17, are

बाहुशोषावबाहुकयोरप्येके वदन्त्यंसयोरन्तरे।

(सु०शा०, 8/17)

Bahushoshavbahukayorapyeke vadantyansayorantare

(Su. Sharir, 8/17)

Puncture and Moxibustion of Pittashay 21 (GB21) which is located in the centre of the shoulder.

See following points also.

Laghvantra 11, 12, 13 (SI 11, 12, 13)
Vrihadantra 16 (LI 16)
Mutrashay 10, 11 (UB 10, 11)

Apasmar (Epilepsy): Location of points as mentioned in *Su. Sharir,* 8/17, are:

हनुसन्धिमध्यगतामपस्मारे।

(सु०शा०, 8/17)

Hanusandhimadhyagatamapasmare

(Su. Sharir, 8/17)

The points for Apasmar are located at the centre of the mandible i.e., Artavnadi 24 (Ren 24).

Puncture as well as Agnikarm (Moxa)

Unmad: See for details, *Su. Sharir,* 8/17:

शंखकेशान्त सन्धिगतामुरोऽपाङ्गललाटेषु चोन्मादे।

(सु०शा०, 8/17)

Shankhkeshant sandhigatamuroapanglalateshu chonmade

(Su. Sharir, 8/17)

The curative points for Unmad are:

1. Shankh Marm
2. Keshant ie Utkshep Marm
3. Ur ie Ren 13, 14, 15. (Artav Nadi)
4. Apang - Pittashay1, Shleshmashay 23 (GB1, Sj23) ?
5. Lalat- Sthapni i.e. Extra

***Method of stimulation*:** Agnikarm (Moxa) is best.

Tritiyak Jvar: (Tertian Malaria): The curative points as given in *Su. Sharir,* 8/17, are:

त्रिकसंधिमध्यगतां तृतीयके

(सु०शा०, 8/17)

Triksandhimadhyagatam triteeyake

(Su. Sharir, 8/17)

According to above shlok the curative points are:
Shukra nadi 13, 14 (DU 13, 14)
Mutrashay 12, 13 (UB 12, 13) of both sides

Method of stimulation:

Siravedhan 0.2 - 0.3 inch and Agnikarm (Moxibustion).

Chaturthak Jvar: (Quartian Malaria): Shlok 8/17, of *Su. Sharir* further indicates curative points.

अधः स्कंधसंधि गतामन्यतर पार्श्वसंस्थितां चतुर्थके।

(सु०शा०, 8/17)

Adhah skandh sandhi gatamanyatar parshvasansthitam chaturthake

(Su.Sharir, 8/17)

The Curative points are:
Shukra nadi 11 (DU 11)
Mutrashay 11 (UB 11)

Jihva Rog and Dant Rog: Acharya suggests:

जिह्वारोगेष्वधोजिह्वायां दन्तव्याधिषु च।

(सु०शा० 8/17)

Jihvarogeshvadhojihvayam dantvyadhishu ch.

(Su. Sharir, 8/17)

For the diseases of the tongue and teeth, puncture the veins under the tongue until bleeding occurs. (This is an extra point named as extra 10).

For Jihvarog see *Sushrut Nidan Mukhrog Nidan.*

Indications:
Stomatitis, Glossitis, Excessive salivation, Infection of the salivary glands, swelling in Gums. Dant-vyadhi includes diseases of root of the tooth which includes diseases of gums. They are fifteen in number. Another diseases of tooth itself are eight in number according to sushrut.

Talu Rog: Sushrut describes nine varieties of Talu Rog, Palate diseases including Tonsilitis, Uvulitis etc. (see *Su. Nidan,* 16/40).

The curative points are:

तालुनि तालव्येषु

(सु०शा०, 8/17)

Taluni talavyeshu

(Su. Sharir, 8/17)

Puncture at the centre of the palate (Siravedh) as well as rub dry salt powder or rub with a specific mixture of following drugs : Black pepper, Atis, Patha, Vach, Kuth, Shyonak, Lavan and honey.

Karna Pida and Karna Rog: For these diseases, Sushrut identifies puncturing points:

कर्णयोरुपरि समन्तात् कर्णशूले तद्रोगेषु च।

(सु०शा०, 8/17)

Karnayorupari samantat karnshule tadrogeshu ch.

(Su. Sharir 8/17)

For the diseases of ear, suppurative otitis media, earache and other ear diseases puncture the points around the ear namely:

Shleshmashay 17, 18, 19 (Sj 17, 18, 19)
Pittashay 2, 10, 17 (GB 2, 10, 17)

Depth for puncture 0.2-0.5 inch. Agnikarm (moxibustion) can be done.

Nasa Rog: For the disease, refer to *Su. Sharir* 8/17:

गन्धाग्रहणे नासारोगेषु च नासाग्रे।

(सु०शा०, 8/17)

Gandhagrahane nasarogeshu ch nasagre

(Su. Sharir, 8/17)

In the diseases of nose and Anosmia prick tip of the nose. The point is Shukra nadi 25 (Du 25).

See also fan Marm in the previous chapters.

Timir Rog, Akshipak: Acharya in *Uttartantra* explains the points of diseases:

तिमिराक्षिपाकप्रभृतिष्वक्ष्यामयेषूपनासिके
ललाट्यामपाङ्गयां वा।।

Timirakshipakprabhritishvakshyamayeshupanasike
lalatyamapangyam va.

In Timir Rog (Diseases of Retina- Dristigat rog) and Akshipak (suppurative conditions of eye), puncture the Siras near the nose Mutrashay 1, 2 (UB1, 2) and lalat Pittashay 14 (GB14) and Apang Pittashay1, Shleshmashay 23 (GB1, Sj 23). For further details see *Sushrut Uttartantra,* seventh chapter.

Acharya Sushrut further advises puncturing of the above mentioned Siras in Sirorog and Adhimanth (Glaucoma like conditions).

GLOSSARY

Adhah	: Downward, below
Adhah Kaya Shosh	: Atrophy of lower half of body
Adhimanth	: Severe pain and irritation of the eyes causing severe headache in half of head with other characteristic signs.
Adhoga	Goes downward as Apan vayu
Adrisht Karm	All physiological actions inside the body
Agneya	Hot and dry in nature
Agnikarm	Hot treatment (Moxibustion)
Akšhi	Eye
Alpa shukrata	Oligospermia
Andhya	Blindness
Angasad	Exhaustion of a body part or body
Angul	Finger (unit of measurement)
Anguli	Finger
Angushth	Toe
Anushna shit	Neither hot nor cold
Apan vayu	One of the five types of vayu mainly having expulsion action
Arasgrahita	Tastelessness
Ardh	Half
Artav nadi	Female dominating channel (Ren channel)
Asammoh	Calmness, deliberateness
Ashmari	Calculus
Ashukriya	Quickness
Asthi	Bone
Asthi shosh	Mere bone, fleshless bone, shrunken bone, osteoporosis.
Asved	Not perspiring
Avedhya	Should not be pierced
Badhiryam	Deafness
Bahvah svapshoshou	Numbness and atrophy of upper extremity

Bhru	:	Eyebrow
Bhrupucchant	:	Lateral end of eyebrow
Chaturvidh Anna	:	Four types of food which we take
Dah	:	Dah kriya (heat treatment)
Dahet	:	Agni dahet (Moxibustion)
Dhanvantari	:	Great Shalya Chikitsak of ancient India, teacher of sushrut
Dharan	:	Maintaining, preserving
Drishti	:	Sight
Dvividh veerya	:	Two types of active principles ushna (hot) sheet (cold)
Gandh	:	Smell
Ghran	:	Nose
Greeva	:	Neck
Gud	:	Anal area
Gulph desh	:	Area of ankle joint
Guru	:	Heavy
Hast	:	Hand
Heen rup	:	Deficient in form or beauty, defective appearance
Him	:	Snow, cold
Jangha	:	Shanks
Jihva	:	Tongue
Kakpad	:	The mark of a crows foot, the claw of crow
Kalantar	:	After sometime
Kalantar pranhar	:	Fatal after sometime
Kanth Nadi	:	Trachea
Kaph vaha	:	Kaph bearing or carrying
Karn	:	ear
Karn shool	:	earache
Kasa shvasa	:	Cough and breathing trouble
Kashay	:	Taste of astringent action
Kati	:	the hip, the loins
Khanj	:	Lameness
Koshth	:	Torso
Kshar	:	Alkali prepared by burning selected herbs and used for cauterization
Kuni	:	Lameness
Kutharika	:	Broad edge cutting instrument having the shape of axe
Kunth or Kunthata	:	Maimed (handicapped related with hand)

Lalat : Forehead
Lepan : The act of anointing
Lohitpoorn : Filled with blood
Madhur : Sweet
Madhye : In between (in the centre)
Manibadh : Area of wrist joint
Mans : Flesh, muscles
Maranam : Death
Marg : way, rout
Medhra : Penis
Mokha tree : A tree which is burnt to make Ash and used to prepare Kshar (Alkaline property)
Mook : Dumb
Mriyate : To death
Mukh : Opening
Murdhni : Apex of head (in the apex Adhipati and Simant Marm reside)
Mutra : Urine
Mutrashay : Urinary bladder
Nirsan : To excrete
Pad : Foot
Pakshaghat : Paralysis of one side
Pakvashay : The seat of digested food
Panch Bhoutik : Made from five elements Akash, Vayu, Tej, Jal, Prithvi
Pandu : Dusty pale, anaemic, yellowish white, jaundiced
Pani : Hand
Param sukshma : Ultramicroscopic
Parshni : The heel
Parshva : Sides, flank, the outer sides of ribs
Payu : Anal orifice
Pishitam : Fresh living flesh
Pitta : One of the three humours
Pittashay : Seat of pitta
Pittavaha : Pitta bearing or carrying
Prabhed : Spliting, piercing, cutting through
Pran : Ras (living factor, pulsating) chinese call it Qi
Pravat : High speed atmospheric air, windy weather
Pran Vayu : One of the five types of Vayu

Pratibaddh : Joints
Prishtha : Back
Prishtha vansh : Vertebral column (the backbone)
Purish : Excreta (stool)
Purush sangyak : Male variety (Yang)
Puy : Pus
Rakta : Fourth humour of Sushrut
Raktashay : Seat of Rakt
Raktavaha : Rakta bearing or carrying
Ras : Essential juice of body, the finest essence of four types of food which we take flows through Dhamanis (channels). This is ultramicroscopic live force which is not detectable in cadavre. According to Sushrut an uninterrupted circulation of Ras is responsible for a good health and any obstacle in the circulation results in disease. The disease is cured if the path of circulation of Ras is revived.
Romkup : Hair follicles
Roop : Shape, to view
Ruja : Pain
Rujakar : Related with pain
Sadya pranhar : Instant death
Sahastra : Thousands of
Sakthi : Lower extremity
Sakthi Shosh : Atrophy of muscles as well as other tissues of lower extremity
Sandhi : Junction, joint, containing a junction or tract from one to the other
Sandhan : To join
Sankochyet : To constrict
Sannipat : Falling in or down together, meeting point
Santarpan : Satiating, feeding
Shabd : Sound, voice
Shadras : Six types of rasas madhur (sweet), amla (sugar), lavan (salt), Katu (pungent), tikta (bitter), kashay (astringent)
Shakha : Extremities
Shalaka : Small rod, a probe, needle, pin, arrow head
Shalya 1. Anything tormenting or causing pain

2. Any disease, any extraneous substance lodged in the body and causing pain e.g. a splinter, pin, stone, fetus and as a branch of medical science to the extraction of above things. 3. Any disease or anything disturbing psychosomatically 4. Javelin, spear, arrow, pointed pin 5. Used in double sense, one for disease and one for instrument.

Shandhya : Impotency

Shankh Pradesh : Temporal area of head

Shastra taikshnya : Sharpness of instruments

Shat : Hundreds of

Sheet : Cool

Shonit : Blood

Shoph : Swelling

Shorya : Courage

Shroni : The hip, loins

Shrot : Ear

Shukra nadi : Male dominating channel (Du-channel)

Sira : Ends, Heads, A stream

Siravyadhan : Therapeutic puncture (Acupuncture)

Skandan : Clotting

Snayu : Ligament, tendon, muscle, nerve, vein

Snehadi : Oil etc.

Snehan : Oleation (anointing). This is a specific preoperative procedure of Panchkarm in which the internal or external application of oils is performed.

Snigdh : Sticky, smooth

Somya : Soft and cool in nature

Son point : Son points are having reducing effect. This is based on Pancha-Mahabhoot theory and used when Svastic yantras are used. Each Dhamani has a mother (Reinforcing) and a Son (Reducing) point. It works under the principle of: 1. *Tatra svayoni vardhananyev pratikarah (Su. Sutra 15/8)*. It means that when Dosh shows reducing sign then reinforce it. 2. *Doshah ksheena vrinhayitavyah, kupita prashamayitavyah, vriddha nirhartavyah, sama paripalya iti siddhantah (Su. Chikitsa 33/3)*

	This indicates that keep doshas in equilibrium by reducing or reinforcing method.
Stabdh bahuta	Numbness of upper extremity
Stabdh sakthita	Numbness of lower extremity
Stan	Breast
Stan choochuk	Nipple
Stri Sangyak	Female Variety (Yin)
Sushrut	Amongst one of the learned disciple of Dhanvantari
Swapanital Kunchit Sammit	The area formed while contracting the palm (2 inches in diameter)
Svarvaikrit	Hoarseness of voice
Svedan	This is a specific preoperative procedure of Panchkarm in which heat or specially medicated steam is used
Tarpayati	Satiating, feeding, nourishing
Tiryag	Goes transverse
Trik	Joints of three bones sacroiliac as well as cervico scapular joint
Trishna	Thirst
Ubhayatah	Both sides
Udar	Abdomen
Upastha	External genitalia
Upghata	Damage, violation
Urdhvaga	Goes upwards, pran
Urdhva jatru	Above clavicle
Uru	Thigh
Ushn	Hot
Va	or
Vaikalya	Imperfection, defectiveness
Vaksh	Chest, torso
Varch	Faecal matter (stool)
Vardhayati	Causing to increase
Vat	Gaseous matters
Vat	One of the three humours
Vataj	Originated from vayu humour
Vatashay	The seat of vayu
Vat vaha	Vat bearing or carrying
Vayavya	Related or belonging to the vayu
Vedhan	Puncturing, piercing, penetration
Veerya	Active principle
Vepathu	Quivering, trembling, tremor

Vidah	:	Burning
Visra	:	Smelling musty or of raw meat
Vivarna	:	Change in colour
Vran	:	A wound, sore, ulcer, abscess, tumour, cancer, boil, scar, Cicatrix, crack
Vriksha	:	Tree
Vrishan	:	Scrotum
Yakrit	:	Liver
Yapan	:	To extract out the disease, treatment of a disease, prolonging or supporting life.
Yav	:	Size of barley grain

Bibliography

Essentials of Chinese Acupuncture, Foreign Language Press, Beijing.

Harrison's Principles of Internal Medicine, 1978.

Parishadyam Shabdarth Shariram.

M. Monier-Williams, *Sanskrit English Dictionary,* Motilal Banarsidass, Delhi, 1999.

Vaman Shivram Apte, *Sanskrit Hindi Kosh,* Oriental Book Centre, Delhi, 1997.

Dr. Ambikadatt Shastri (Ed.), *Sushrut Samhita,* Chowkhamba Sanskrit Sansthan, Varanasi, 1985.

Atridev (Ed.), *Sushrut Samhita,* Motilal Banarasidass, Delhi, 1998.

Sushrut and Huang ti nei Ching, Dr. R.L. Shah.

INDEX

FIGURE INDEX